POWER OVER CANCER

Vernon Coleman

BOOKS BY VERNON COLEMAN

The Medicine Men (1975)
Paper Doctors (1976)
Everything You Want To Know About Ageing (1976)
Stress Control (1978)
The Home Pharmacy (1980)
Aspirin or Ambulance (1980)
Face Values (1981)
Guilt (1982)
The Good Medicine Guide (1982)
Stress And Your Stomach (1983)
Bodypower (1983)
An A to Z Of Women's Problems (1984)
Bodysense (1984)
Taking Care Of Your Skin (1984)
Life Without Tranquillisers (1985)
High Blood Pressure (1985)
Diabetes (1985)
Arthritis (1985)
Eczema and Dermatitis (1985)
The Story Of Medicine (1985)
Natural Pain Control (1986)
Mindpower (1986)
Addicts and Addictions (1986)
Dr Vernon Coleman's Guide To Alternative Medicine (1988)
Stress Management Techniques (1988)
Overcoming Stress (1988)
Know Yourself (1988)
The Health Scandal (1988)
The 20 Minute Health Check (1989)
Sex For Everyone (1989)
Mind Over Body (1989)
Eat Green Lose Weight (1990)
Toxic Stress (1991)
Why Animal Experiments Must Stop (1991)
The Drugs Myth (1992)

Why Doctors Do More Harm Than Good (1993)
Stress and Relaxation (1993)
Complete Guide to Sex (1993)
How to Conquer Backache (1993)
How to Conquer Arthritis (1993)
Betrayal of Trust (1994)
Know Your Drugs (1994)
Food for Thought (1994)
The Traditional Home Doctor (1994)
I Hope Your Penis Shrivels Up (1994)
People Watching (1995)
Relief from IBS (1995)
The Parent's Handbook (1995)
Oral Sex: Bad Taste And Hard To Swallow (1995)
Why Is Pubic Hair Curly? (1995)
Men in Dresses (1996)

novels
The Village Cricket Tour (1990)
The Bilbury Chronicles (1992)
Bilbury Grange (1993)
Mrs Caldicot's Cabbage War (1993)
The Man Who Inherited a Golf Course (1993)
Bilbury Revels (1994)
Deadline (1994)

short stories
Bilbury Pie (1995)

on cricket
Thomas Winsden's Cricketing Almanack (1983)
Diary Of A Cricket Lover (1984)

as Edward Vernon
Practice Makes Perfect (1977)
Practise What You Preach (1978)

Getting Into Practice (1979)
Aphrodisiacs - An Owners Manual (1983)
Aphrodisiacs - An Owners Manual (Turbo Edition) (1984)
The Complete Guide To Life (1984)

as Marc Charbonnier
Tunnel (novel 1980)

with Dr Alan C Turin
No More Headaches (1981)

with Alice
Alice's Diary (1989)
Alice's Adventures (1992)

POWER OVER CANCER

Vernon Coleman

European Medical Journal

Published by European Medical Journal, Publishing House, Trinity Place, Barnstaple, Devon EX32 9HJ, England

First published in the United Kingdom by the European Medical Journal in 1996.

ISBN: 1 898947 98 8

A catalogue record for this book is available from the British Library.

Printed and bound by: J.W. Arrowsmith, Bristol

Dedication

To Thomasina:
A loving, loyal friend and a good companion; a constant joy and an ever present assistant

And to Alice:
Who will forever have a place in my heart and who is missed today just as much as she ever was, and who will be missed tomorrow just as much as she is today

CONTENTS

FORWARD

I started to research this subject for my own benefit. Since qualifying as a doctor just over two decades ago I have read much conflicting information about cancer and I wanted to find out the truth for myself. I knew that I should follow a diet that contained natural fibre and that was low in fat but I wanted to know more. I wanted to make sure that I ate a diet that would give me the best possible chance of avoiding cancer. I wanted to find out what researchers had discovered in the last two decades.

The more I studied, and the more I searched for information, the more convinced I became that the truth about the links between food and cancer had been deliberately suppressed by industries determined to continue to sell their existing products (whatever the human cost might be), by politicians committed to supporting those industries and by a medical profession which has become a pawn of the pharmaceutical industry.

You may be as surprised as I was to find that the knowledge that there is a link between food and cancer is not new. Way back in January 1892 Scientific American magazine reported: 'cancer is most frequent among those branches of the human race where carnivorous habits prevail'. Even before that, in 1804, J Abernethy, in 'Surgical Observations on Tumours' reported on the effectiveness of a vegetarian diet as a treatment for cancer. Indeed, according to a report published in 1988 by the United States Department of Health and Human Services, called 'The Surgeon General's Report on Nutrition and Health', diet has been suspected as a cause of cancer since the disease was recognised in the first century A.D. Empirical evidence was first reported in 1913 and studies were published over half a century ago demonstrating the links between food and cancer. In 1933 researchers suggested that wholemeal bread and cruciferous vegetables helped to protect against cancer and in 1940 insurance company records suggested that over-weight individuals were more likely to develop cancer than normal or underweight people. This research led to plenty of experiments involving animals (lots of researchers altered the dietary habits of animals to find out whether or not they were more or less likely to develop cancer) but no one seemed too concerned to apply the knowledge that had been obtained from a study of human beings to human beings, and little effort was made to conduct further epidemiological studies.

In 'Nutrition and Health', the report published in 1988 by the United States Surgeon General, a table was published suggesting that diet could be responsible for up to 70 per cent of all cancers - with a (conservative) 'best estimate' suggesting that diet was responsible for 35 per cent of all cancers.

The Surgeon General suggested five possible mechanisms to explain the 'observed association between diet, digestive processes and cancer'. These were:

1. The presence of carcinogens in food. These could be present naturally, could be contaminants or could be formed as a result of cooking or preserving the food.

2. Carcinogens within the body might be activated or deactivated by something in the diet. For example, the beta carotene present in some foods may slow down or block potentially cancer inducing processes.

3. Carcinogens may be formed within the body. For example, naturally produced bile acids, excreted to help deal with consumed fats, may be converted into tumour producing chemicals by bacteria which live in the colon. The bacteria may be affected by diet.

4. The cancer process may be enhanced by some foods (for example fats) or may be inhibited by some foods (for example, vitamin A).

5. An imbalance of nutrients may impair the immunity of the body and may, therefore, affect the ability of the body to defend itself - either by repairing damaged DNA or by rejecting malignant cells.

I had not intended to write this book when I started my researches. But having discovered what I have discovered I had no choice but to publish a book containing my findings.

Although the bulk of this book deals with food (partly because food is the main cause of cancer and partly because there is more confusion and misinformation about the links between food and cancer than there is, say, about the links between tobacco and cancer) I have also included information about most of the other well known or suspected links. I do not, however, suggest that the list of possible causes of cancer in this book is comprehensive. I have dealt with the causes which attract most attention and which I regard both as being of most significance and easiest to do something about.

Cancer inducing chemicals are all around us - in air polluted with tobacco smoke and chemicals, in food and in the chemical products with which our homes are crammed. Our bodies are constantly producing potentially cancerous cells. We can help to protect ourselves against cancer by avoiding the obvious carcinogens (such as tobacco, fat and meat) but we can also build up our defence systems, and protect ourselves against cancer, by eating the right foods.

Finally, I think it is appropriate to point out that my own eating habits certainly follow the advice in this book. In other words 'I practise what I preach'! I believe that the earlier you adopt the eating habits recommended in this book the lower your cancer risk will be. But I also believe that it is never too late to change.

Vernon Coleman 1995

PREFACE

Cancer is not a single disease. It is a word which describes a great many quite different diseases. The one thing they all have in common is that there is an uncontrolled and disorderly growth of abnormal cells. It is quite normal for cells to grow and to reproduce. Every minute, in every human body, an astonishing ten million cells divide. Usually everything goes well. The cells divide in the right way and at the right time. But when a cell becomes a 'cancer cell' it grows and divides at an abnormally rapid rate. These abnormal 'cancer cells' destroy or push aside the normal, functioning cells. If the 'cancer cells' are not stopped they may spread to other parts of the body and take up residence in other, different organs. 'Cancer cells' may be carried around the body through the blood vessels or the lymph channels. When a cancer spreads and appears in another part of the body the new growths are known as metastases. Cancer can also spread by 'crab-like' outgrowths (hence the name 'cancer'). It is now widely accepted that many of the cancers which most commonly occur develop because outside substances trigger some sort of reaction - and cancer development - in the body. This book is much concerned with those 'triggers'.

Cancer is not the unknown, dark shrouded mystery killer which it is often thought to be. We do not know enough to recommend a diet which will enable all individuals to avoid all food related cancers. But we know enough to make a difference. If we make the decision to avoid those foods and other substances which research has shown can lead to the development of cancer, and to eat those foods which can strengthen our defences against cancer, then I believe that we can dramatically influence our susceptibility to the disease.

It is fairly wide known, I think, that cigarettes, sunshine, asbestos and X rays cause cancer. But it is less widely known that fatty foods and meat cause cancer. And it is less well known that fibre and green vegetables help protect against cancer.

People get cancer through bad luck and inherited susceptibilities. But they also get it through ignorance - ignorance which has been deliberately sustained through commercial greed and political expediency. When businessmen, politicians and doctors know how to prevent 80 per cent of cancers but do nothing it is difficult to avoid the conclusion that those cancer deaths are deliberate. Eight out of ten people who die from cancer have effectively been murdered in cold blood. It is difficult to avoid the conclusion that cancer is now often a disease of choice - but the choice is made for us by those whose sense of responsibility does not match their authority. For too many people the choice is made by politicians, businessmen and doctors who do not understand that with knowledge comes responsibility.

In the 'Proceedings of the Nutrition Society' in 1990, Sir Richard Doll said: 'There is now uniform agreement among oncologists that the incidence of cancer is determined, in large part, by factors in the environment and aspects of behaviour that are capable of modification or avoidance.'

For decades much of the international 'cancer industry' has been devoted to finding magical 'cures' for cancer - with little useful effect. But since many of the causes of cancer are known my aim in this book is quite simply to explain those causes and to tell you how you can best cut your own risk of developing cancer substantially.

Changing large organisations can take decades and generations. I have absolutely no doubt that in a few decades time eating meat, drinking milk and smoking tobacco will be regarded as bizarre and reckless practices. Our descendants will not understand why we exposed ourselves to such unnecessary risks. But it will take time for those changes to take place. There are laboratories to dismantle and companies to close down; butchers' shops to shut and farmers to direct away from animal farming and towards the growing of healthy crops. With so many vested interests to oppose all this will take a long time.

But you do not have to wait for the authorities to tell you what to eat and what to avoid eating. You do not have to wait for the food companies to start selling foods that will limit your chances of developing cancer. You don't have to wait for the cancer industry to turn its attention away from pointless and misleading animal experiments and start telling you what to eat to reduce your cancer risk. You can take action now. This book will tell you how you can help yourself reduce your cancer risk by up to 80 per cent. Since we know what causes around 80 per cent of cancers it is clear that we also know how to avoid 80 per cent of cancers. I cannot and do not guarantee that you won't get cancer if you follow the advice in this book. But I do firmly believe that your chances of developing cancer will be significantly lower than it will be if you take no action to protect yourself. And I also believe that if you do develop cancer then the advice in this book will improve your chances of fighting your cancer and winning.

Vernon Coleman, 1995

PART ONE
THE CANCER INDUSTRY: MISDIRECTED
AND INEFFECTIVE

CHAPTER ONE
THE WAR AGAINST CANCER

Cancer is, along with heart disease and stroke, one of the three big killers of our time. But cancer is the killer that frightens people most. The very word is so emotive that most doctors try not to use it when talking to patients. Instead of talking of cancer they talk of 'tumours' and 'growths'. They know that cancer is something most people don't even like to talk about.

Cancer of the colon is a much bigger killer than AIDS but you won't see many show business fund raisers being organised to help colon cancer sufferers in the way that money is raised to help AIDS sufferers (although money is raised - in vast quantities - to help pay for the salaries and expenses of researchers looking for a cure for cancer).

Until it touches them or someone in their family most people try not to think about cancer. When they see a collecting tin for a cancer charity they may pop in a few coins in the belief that by making a donation to a cancer charity they are helping to conquer the disease. Putting money into a cancer charity collecting tin is like throwing coins into a wishing well; it is the twentieth century equivalent of a good luck charm.

In order to ensure that money continues to pour in the cancer industry must persuade potential contributors and supporters that it is making progress in the fight against cancer. Like all large organisations the cancer industry needs a vast quantity of money just to remain in business; there are salaries to be paid, rents and rates to be paid, electricity bills to be paid, advertising and public relations departments to pay for and so on.

To help in this aim the huge worldwide cancer industry must frequently release news about exciting new cancer remedies. Some of these widely promoted new treatments are in the early stages of being tested on human patients, some are not yet being tested on humans but are promoted as the new 'wonder' cure for cancer on the basis of animal experiments, and some are talked about as new 'breakthroughs' largely or even exclusively on the basis of a scientist's theory or hypothesis. These news stories may raise hopes falsely and they certainly distract attention and finance from those areas which really need it (the prevention of cancer and the care of those who have cancer) but they serve the purpose: they raise money for the cash hungry cancer industry.

When someone rattles a collecting tin in front of you and tells you that they need just a few more pence in order to continue with their breakthrough research it is difficult to say 'no'. It is hardly surprising that the worldwide cancer industry's income continues to grow at a quite phenomenal rate.

But has the cancer industry really made any noticeable progress in the fight against cancer? I don't think so. The mortality figures show that more people are dying from cancer now than were a generation ago. One in three people already have, or will develop, cancer. According to journal 'The Sciences' (published by the New York Academy of Sciences) the American Cancer Society has estimated that over half a million Americans were killed by cancer in 1994 alone - twice as many as were killed in the Second World War. Figures from around the world show that the picture is much the same everywhere.

In the nineteenth century cancer was a relatively uncommon disease. According to Garrison's 'History of Medicine' it showed an 'alarming increase' in the early part of the twentieth century. Today, as I have already mentioned, cancer is firmly positioned (along with heart disease and stroke) as one of the three big 'killers' of the westernised world. The fact that the incidence of cancer has increased dramatically during the 20th century confirms, in my opinion, the view that cancer is, to a large extent, a man-made disease, created largely by our changing diet and our addiction to tobacco. In America it has been estimated that around $110 billion a year is spent on cancer. That is more than ten per cent of American's entire health care bill. But, in America, during the last fifteen years or so the incidence of cancer has steadily risen as has the number of people dying of cancer.

Writing in the European Medical Journal in Winter 1993 Dr Jack Tropp pointed out that 'despite the billions of dollars spent each year for cancer research and treatment, using the traditional methods of choice: surgery, chemotherapy and radiation therapy, in the overall picture nothing has changed in the mortality rates in the last thirty five years.'

Scientists who have assessed the value of the war against cancer agree that we are losing the fight and that there is no evidence to suggest that decades of expensive research have had much, if any, effect on the most fundamental measure of success or failure - death. In areas where cancer has become more amenable to treatment, or now takes fewer lives, it is usually changes in life style which are responsible - not discoveries made in the laboratory.

In my view, the effort, the money, and all the misguided hope and faith that has been poured into cancer research by the international cancer industry simply hasn't worked. And there are, I believe, several reasons why those fighting the war against cancer are losing. In my book 'Paper Doctors' (published in 1977) I complained that: 'Medical researchers involved in publicly or charitably financed cancer research persist in looking for the 'magical cure'. Much laboratory work has been started on the mistaken assumption that there is one disease called 'cancer' and that there will be a 'cure' which will enable doctors to treat all the patients suffering with cancer. Many projects have been funded because organisers (both qualified and lay) have believed that they might solve the problem of cancer once and for all to the well publicised credit of everyone concerned. Much money has undoubtedly been wasted on research which has duplicated work done elsewhere and which has moved in directions unlikely ever to prove of practical benefit.'

These complaints, made nearly twenty years ago, are now frequently echoed by other observers. In the March/April 1995 issue of 'The Sciences' Robert N Proctor, associate professor of the history of science at Pennsylvania State University and author of 'Cancer Wars: How Politics Shapes What We Know and Don't Know About Cancer', pointed out that: 'Part of the problem lies in the very belief that a single, universal cure can be found.'

CHAPTER TWO
WOMEN GOLFERS AND BREAST CANCER

B reast cancer is one of the most constantly publicised and most greatly feared forms of cancer. Because of its very nature it is a type of cancer which arouses much emotion. Newspapers, magazines and medical journals have for decades been full of articles describing new forms of treatment. The medical journal, 'The Lancet', in an editorial, commented that: 'If one were to believe all the media hype, the triumphalism of the profession in published research, and the almost weekly miracle breakthroughs trumpeted by the cancer charities, one might be surprised that women are dying at all from this cancer.'

But women are still dying from breast cancer. Indeed, the overall death rate from breast cancer hasn't changed and isn't changing. Despite all the talk and all the promises the number of women dying from breast cancer hasn't altered. The disease is still as great a killer as it was decades ago. 'In the two short decades since Nixon began shovelling money into the NCI (National Cancer Institute) breast cancer has claimed more U.S. lives than the Vietnam War, the Korean War, World War I and World War II put together,' reported the journal 'Australian Health and Healing'.

The real tragedy is that since 1942 there has been steadily accumulating evidence to show that there is link between breast cancer and dietary fat. I have little doubt that breast cancer could have been turned into a relatively uncommon disease, instead of one of the major killers of women, if politicians and doctors had been prepared to take on the food industry - and force the cancer industry to spread the truth. In Britain around 15,000 women die of breast cancer every year. That is roughly one every half hour. And yet if those women had known which foods to eat - and which to avoid - half of them could still be alive today.

Despite the quantity of epidemiological evidence which is available to show that fat and breast cancer are linked (and I have detailed some of this evidence later in this book) no one really knows the mechanism through which fat causes cancer. One theory is that synthetic chemicals - commonly used in the manufacture of pesticides - concentrate in the fatty tissues of animals. People who then eat animal after animal absorb the synthetic chemicals into their own bodies - and the concentrations of chemicals steady rise. (In an average lifetime a meat eater will consume 36 pigs, 36 sheep, 750 chickens and turkeys and several cows.)

According to the journal 'Australasian Health and Healing' more than 177 organochlorines (synthetic chemicals created when chlorine gas is bonded to carbon-rich organic matter) have been found in the tissues of the general population of the United States and Canada. Organochlorines can cause infertility, birth defects, miscarriages, immune system suppression, metabolic dysfunction, behavioural disorders, hormonal abnormalities and cancer.

These chlorine based compounds can cause cancer in various ways. Some cause cancer directly. Others produce cancers by interfering with or mimicking human hormones. A third group suppress the immune system and then enhance the carcinogenic effect of other chemicals. These chemicals seem to strike first at the reproductive system - which is probably why a heavy fat consumption increases the risk of developing cancers of the breast, prostate, and uterus.

We accept chemicals because they make our life easier and because the big chemical companies have become financially and politically powerful. We assume that they are essential and we assume that they are safe because that is what the big companies tell us. I don't believe they are essential and I certainly don't believe that they are safe.

Here is some of the epidemiological evidence collected by the journal 'Australasian Health and Healing' to support the theory that it is the chemicals in fat which cause cancer:

∗ Women in parts of America which were routinely blanketed with aerial sprayings of the pesticide DDT during the 1950s have one of the highest rates of breast cancer in America.

∗ Female chemical workers who were exposed to high

levels of dioxin in a German pesticide plant had double the cancer mortality rate of the German population - and higher than average rates of breast cancer. A study in America produced similar results.

* Women professional golfers, most of whom played the game every day, have a high rate of breast cancer. It is suspected that these women may have been poisoned by the chemicals with which most golf courses are saturated.

* According to a U.S. Environmental Protection Agency study parts of America with hazardous waste sites were 6.5 times as likely to have a high breast cancer rate than other areas.

* Women who have breast cancer have high blood levels of the chemicals suspected of causing the disease. A study of 229 women from New York City showed that women who developed breast cancer had substantially higher levels of suspected pesticide chemicals.

* During the early 1970s breast cancer rates in Israel were among the highest and fastest rising in the world. In 1978 Israel phased out the use of several suspected pesticides. Doctors noted that the levels of chemicals in breast milk dropped quite quickly. The incidence of breast cancer duly started to fall too.

Despite all this evidence I can't tell you exactly how fat causes cancer. But does the mechanism whereby fat causes cancer really matter? It would, it is true, be nice to know how fat causes cancer. But do we have to know how fat causes cancer before we decide to cut down our fat consumption?

The medical profession, which has largely ignored the existing evidence showing what causes breast cancer, does, of course, remain willing to continue to make money out of 'treating' women who develop breast cancer.

Perhaps the biggest irony of all is the fact that although doctors have widely ignored the available evidence that would have enabled them to protect most of their patients from breast cancer (and, indeed, many other major types of cancer too) they have devised their own high technology form of preventive medicine - the mammogram. It is difficult not to be cynical about this. Teaching women how to reduce their chances of developing breast cancer (and teaching them how to check their own breasts for lumps) would earn the profession very little. So the medical profession - and its companion industries - have introduced a high technology form of cancer detection so that they can make money out of the general anxiety about breast cancer.

In my book 'The Health Scandal' (which was published in 1988 and violently attacked by doctors all over the country - even though some of those who were doing the attacking admitted that they hadn't actually bothered to read it) I objected to mammography screening partly on the grounds that there must surely be risks in having regular X ray examinations (it would, I thought, be hideously, grotesquely ironic if a new technique designed to spot breast cancer at an early stage turned out, twenty years later, to cause breast cancer) and partly on the grounds that a mass breast screening programme simply would not work and would not make a significant difference to the number of women dying of breast cancer because the interval of one year between examinations was too long.

I pointed out that the available evidence showed clearly that self examination was much better and more effective (as well as being considerably cheaper and requiring far less highly trained medical manpower).'A proper educational programme' I wrote, 'designed to teach British women how to examine their breasts properly, would undoubtedly have a dramatic effect on the number of women dying from breast cancer in Britain. It would cost very little and it would produce continuing results. But it would not, of course, provide work for the unwanted radiologists who we are training every year. And it probably wouldn't satisfy the strident spokeswomen who believe that annual screening clinics must be better than regular checks done at home.'

At the time this comment was dismissed as heresy by many in the medical establishment who argued that self screening was useless. But seven years later more doctors began to question the logic of mammography. And by then several studies had suggested that the radiation accumulated through yearly mammograms might actually be causing breast cancer.

The ultimate irony is, perhaps, the fact that the pharmaceutical industry makes billions of dollars selling drugs for the treatment of cancers which some believe may have been created by its billion dollar sister industry: the chemical industry.

Doctors and drug companies and the cancer industry have come together in the belief that the best way to deal with cancer (or to prevent it) is to use drugs.

Consider, for example, the tamoxifen experiment - designed to find out if the drug tamoxifen will protect women from breast cancer.

The drug tamoxifen isn't new. For several years it has been given to women who are suffering from breast cancer and as a treatment for infertility. The risks associated with this drug may be low enough to justify its use when a woman's life is threatened because she already has cancer but just look at the possible side effects which may be associated with tamoxifen: hot flushes, vaginal bleeding, gastro-intestinal pain, light headedness, skin rash, cataracts, fluid retention, and endometrial carcinoma.

I suppose the politicians and scientists who are in charge of this extraordinary trial may claim that women won't mind feeling light headed, developing a skin rash and cataracts and suffering from hot flushes and vaginal bleeding if there is a chance that they will be less likely to get breast cancer but what about that last hazard: endometrial carcinoma? Endometrial carcinoma is cancer of the uterus!

So, according to the existing information we already have about this drug we know that there is a possible risk that it may cause cancer of the uterus. And governments around the world have given researchers approval to give it to thousands of perfectly healthy women to see if it stops them getting breast cancer.

What sort of inspired lunacy is this?

These healthy women - some of them still in their 30s - will be given the drug to take for several years.

Those who are organising the trial are also ignoring evidence showing that tamoxifen causes liver cancer in rats and gonadal cancer in mice. As I have been arguing for years animal experiments cannot be used to predict what will happen when a drug is given to human patients. (Though some readers may, like me, find it a little difficult to understand why the cancer industry still supports animal experiments when it is insisting that the tamoxifen experiments on animals be ignored so that they can go ahead with this human experiment!).

If those who are organising the trial are satisfied with the results doctors around the world will, presumably, be encouraged to prescribe tamoxifen on a regular basis for millions of healthy women. The drug could quickly become one of the most profitable pharmacological products ever marketed.

CHAPTER THREE
ANIMAL EXPERIMENTS: MORE HARM THAN GOOD

Raising money for cancer research is now big business. But it is a business that has, if you assess its effectiveness critically, surely been a dismal failure. One of the main reasons why the cancer industry has failed is because it has concentrated too much of its massive effort on animal experiments. Millions of pounds have, for example, been spent on giving cancer to animals - when it has for years been widely appreciated that the cancers animals get are quite different to the cancers people get.

Animal experiments are cheap, relatively easy to perform, do not require great skills, and tend to produce some sort of result very quickly. Cancer research workers often work together with big drug companies which love animal experiments for their double edged value. If an experiment on a group of animals shows that a drug does not harm those particular animals then the drug company will use the evidence to ensure that the drug is given a clean bill of health around the world. But if an experiment on a group of animals shows that the drug does harm those particular animals the drug company will ignore the evidence on the grounds that animals are different to people - and that the results are, therefore, of no significance. As the American Committee on Diet, Nutrition and Cancer (of the U.S. National Research Council) pointed out in 'Diet, Nutrition and Cancer' (published by the National Academy Press): 'animals are not human, and the etiology of the cancers they develop may not duplicate that for cancers in humans.' The United States Surgeon General has pointed out: 'an important weakness is that virtually all animal studies test single, genetically uniform (inbred) strains of one or two nonhuman species under highly uniform conditions of diet, temperature, stress, exposure to infectious diseases etc'.

Cancer researchers frequently claim that if animal experiments are banned they will never be able to find a cure for cancer. The choice, they say to those who dare to question what they do, is simple: the lives of a few animals (since animal researchers around the world kill around one thousand animals every thirty seconds this is something of an under-statement) or the lives of your children. This crude and, sadly, often effective blackmail (which I have previously described as a form of intellectual terrorism) presupposes that cancer researchers are eventually going to find a 'cure' for cancer - indeed, it assumes, quite illogically, that there can ever be a single cure for the two hundred quite different diseases which make up the group of illnesses we know as 'cancer'. There is no evidence at all to suggest that this is an accurate presupposition.

On the contrary the evidence clearly shows that animal experiments are a complete waste of time, that animal experiments have never led to any useful breakthroughs and that they are never likely to lead to any useful breakthroughs.

Animals get cancer, it is true, but the cancers they get are quite different to the types of cancer which affect human beings. Moreover, animals respond quite differently to the various types of treatment which are available. The results animal researchers obtain are totally without value. The total uncertainty makes the whole business valueless.

Instead of helping doctors find a cure for cancer those scientists who do experiments on animals have held back medical progress and have been responsible for much pain and distress and hundreds of thousands of unnecessary deaths.

A standard test used on rats gives results which can be accurately applied to human beings just 38 per cent of the time. This means that 62 per cent of the time the results obtained through animal experiments are wrong. Since tossing a coin would give a long term 50 per cent chance of accuracy it would clearly be quicker, more effective, more efficient and cheaper for these scientists to spend their working days sitting around tossing coins to assess the safety of chemicals. ('Heads! Yes! We can give this to patients! Tails! No! Patients can't take that one.')

But, in political and financial terms, tossing a coin would certainly not be as useful as using animals. Consider tobacco, for example. The link between tobacco and cancer was identified many years ago by doctors whose observations and research work had involved human patients. But long after doctors had established the link between tobacco and cancer in humans animal researchers were still forcing dogs to smoke and painting tobacco tar on the backs of mice in attempts to show whether or not there was a laboratory link between tobacco and cancer. Politicians who wanted to avoid taking action against the wealthy and big tax paying tobacco companies (the U.S. government receives more than $13 billion a year in tobacco tax) were able to do so on the grounds that they were still awaiting laboratory confirmation of the link between tobacco and cancer. Decades of vague, inconclusive and contradictory results have enabled the world's tobacco industry to keep selling a product which is responsible for approximately one third of all cancer deaths and which, over the years, must have been responsible for more deaths, disease and misery than any other product ever invented.

Using animals to test new anti-cancer drugs is equally absurd. 'Test beds' made of human tissue cells are available. These can be used reliably to test anti-cancer drugs. I cannot see the scientific sense in testing a drug on animals when it can be tested on cells which are identical to those within the patients who will take the drug. (There is, as I have already pointed out, coarse commercial sense in doing such tests on animals. If a test on one species show that a drug is lethal the test can be repeated on another species, and another, and another until a more promising or acceptable result is obtained. The drug can then be launched worldwide as suitable for human patients.)

Animal experiments are useless because animals are completely different to people. According to Dr Irwin Bross, giving evidence to the United States Congress: 'conflicting animal results have often delayed and hampered the war on cancer, they have never produced a single, substantial advance either in the prevention or treatment of human cancer.' The medical journal The Lancet commented that: 'since no animal tumour is closely related to a cancer in human beings an agent which is active in the laboratory may well prove useless clinically.'

CHAPTER FOUR
THE SEARCH FOR A MAGIC CURE

Huge amounts of money have been spent on searching for a 'magic' cure for cancer when cancer is scores of different diseases and it is as unlikely that we are going to find a single cure for all these different diseases as we are to find a single drug that will cure all infections.

Most of the effort expended by the cancer industry has been spent on searching for the ever elusive cure. And yet throughout medical history it has consistently been clear that it is invariably easier and more effective (and, in the long run a great deal cheaper) to prevent illness than it is to try and cure it. The evidence shows quite clearly that any improvements in life expectancy which have taken place in the last few decades have been almost entirely due not to the development of a sophisticated and expensive medical profession or the development of a highly profitable international pharmaceutical industry but to simple improvements in living standards. The enemies of death and disease in the last century have not been doctors and drug companies but (relatively) clean drinking water and better sewage facilities. There has been a modest improvement in life expectancy in the last hundred years but it has been nothing to do drugs or surgery.

(And the improvement has been more modest than most doctors like to admit. Figures for the UK are difficult to get hold of because the British Government traditionally regards every health care statistic as a state secret, to be shared only with the pharmaceutical industry, but figures published by the United States Bureau of Census show that 33 per cent of people born in 1907 could expect to live to the age of 75. Later figures show that 33 per cent of the people born in 1977 could expect to live to the age of 80. Remove the improvements produced by better living conditions, cleaner water supplies, and the reduction in deaths during or just after childbirth and it becomes clear that doctors, drug companies and hospitals cannot possibly have had any useful effect on life expectancy. Indeed, the figures show that there has been an increase in mortality rates among the middle aged and a dramatic increase in the incidence of disorders such as diabetes, arthritis, heart disease and cancer.)

The truth is that the inventor of the flush lavatory has saved a million times more lives than any doctor. It is not the men who discovered antibiotics - and who now prescribe them with such reckless overenthusiasm - whom we should thank for the virtual disappearance of some of the best known killer infectious diseases of the nineteenth century but the men who dug our sewers and laid the first water pipes.

We don't need more money pouring into cancer research because we already know what causes most forms of cancer. According to one honest observer: 'Basic cancer research is an excellent slush fund for molecular biologists but it won't have any impact on cancer'. Cancer is created by chemical pollutants, by unhealthy, fatty, food and by tobacco. Poisoned water supplies, dangerous prescription drugs and the over use of X rays have also contributed to the incidence of cancer.

With immune systems constantly battered by polluted air, adulterated and chemically impregnated food and a constant onslaught from the drugs we buy for ourselves, or allow our doctors to prescribe for us, it is not surprising that increasing numbers of people succumb to one of the many different types of cancer. We know what causes 80 per cent of all cases of cancer! Eight out of ten people who develop cancer could have been saved if money and effort had been put into prevention.

I do not believe that any wonder cure for cancer will come from the 'cancer industry'.But if I had the annual income the cancer industry enjoys I believe that I could turn cancer into a historical oddity within five years.

'Why,' you may ask, 'do the big cancer charities not spend more money on trying to prevent cancer? Why do they spend all their money gambling on the chance of finding a 'cure' when they could save millions of lives simply by using their resources to publicise what we already know?'

To understand the answers to these questions you have to

understand that the cancer research industry is exactly that - an industry. It is a massive, worldwide multi-billion dollar industry which employs hundreds of thousands of scientists and administrators. Sadly, I suspect that for many of these employees the search for a cure for cancer has become the end instead of just the beginning. Much of the cancer industry is run by and for scientific researchers. The cancer industry needs a constant stream of dollars to keep its laboratories running. If the cancer industry spent its income on explaining to people how to avoid cancer there would be little or no place for research laboratories and a great many scientists would be put out of work. Worse still, if the cancer industry reduced the number of people dying of cancer its own income would fall.

Besides, those whose job it is to raise money know that it is far easier to persuade people to put money into a collecting tin if you tell them that they are contributing towards the search for a cure. Persuading people to avoid known causes of cancer is thankless work. Not many people will put money into your collecting tin if you stand on a street corner handing out leaflets containing sensible eating advice. It is much easier to raise money if you talk about new breakthroughs and show photographs of people (preferably children or pretty young women) who are dying of cancer. It is much easier to raise a million dollars for a new piece of machinery than it is to raise a million dollars for a print bill or a television advertising campaign designed to explain to people how they can avoid cancer.

Those who are responsible for raising money for the cancer industry know that it is impossible to personalise a preventive medicine campaign because you can never show a picture of a man, woman or child whose life has been saved by a leaflet. A picture of a child who is dying of cancer and who is waiting for laboratory scientists to find a cure will attract far more public support than an appeal for funds to help save unnamed individuals in the future.

And so it is the scientists searching for laboratory cures who get the big grants and the prestigious awards and who are fussed over and praised by the politicians and the journalists. Scientists who have established links which would enable us to save millions of lives by organising effective prevention programmes are as unlikely to win Nobel prizes as are doctors who devote themselves to teaching the principles of healthy living to millions of people.

My book 'Paper Doctors' (which was published in 1977) contained a whole chapter attacking the cancer industry in some detail. 'According to the International Agency for Research on Cancer 80 per cent of all cancers are environmentally induced,' I wrote. 'The Director of the American National Cancer Institute has publicly stated that he believes that the figure is nearer to 90 per cent. Eric Boyland, for many years Professor of Biochemistry at the Institute of Cancer Research in London, concluded after careful consideration of all the likely causes of cancer that between 85 and 90 per cent of all human tumours are caused by chemicals. According to the 1974/5 Annual Report of the Medical Research Council, 'This statement has never been seriously challenged and the experience and research of the past few years has tended to support this view of cancer."

Further on in the same chapter in 'Paper Doctors' I went on to say: 'If we took the advice given by the experts who quote these figures then we could cut down cancer rates dramatically. However, the emphasis among cancer researchers is very much on finding a cure rather than reducing the incidence of cancer. Since there is so much evidence to show that the causative factors can be controlled (cigarettes cause one third of all cancers in the United Kingdom) that is, to say the least, surprising. There are many explanations for this disastrous misreading of the needs within cancer research. Undoubtedly one important reason is that there are thousands of surgeons, radiologists and radiotherapists (not to mention pure researchers) earning their living from traditional methods of cancer research and control. Public health is not a fashionable speciality within the medical profession: there is no opportunity for private practice and a general lack of financial incentive for brighter physicians to enter this field. And of equal importance perhaps is the fact that industrial pressures all oppose attempts to control the causative factors responsible for the vast majority of cancers.'

'I doubt if you will even think of all this next time you see a stranger shaking a collecting tin at you and asking for a contribution towards cancer research. You, like everyone else, have been lured over the years into believing the claims and promises made by honestly motivated but misdirected cancer researchers. If you really cared about cancer patients you would give your money to a caring organisation or an anti-smoking campaign, taking note of Lord Zuckerman's conclusion in his official Report entitled 'Cancer Research' published in 1972. He wrote that 'a sudden increase in funds for cancer research could not be effectively used' and suggested that money be spent on helping those struggling to look after relatives dying of cancer rather than on more research programmes.'

But those words fell on deaf ears.

In the two decades since 'Paper Doctors' was published the cancer industry has continued to grow. It is now a multi-billion dollar industry. The cancer researchers are still pleading for more money; they are still claiming that if they are given enough money they will be able to find a cure for cancer. It is, they suggest, only a shortage of money which is responsible for the continuing rise in the incidence of cancer deaths. They want to do more animal experiments and they have now devised animals which are genetically bred to develop cancer.

Cancer industry employees say they want to know 'how' cancer develops. They don't seem to understand that the 'how' is not important. It would be nice to know the 'how'. But it is the 'why' which matters. And we already know why cancer is a major killer.

By insisting on finding the 'how' the cancer industry is playing right into the hands of the industries which are responsible for much cancer. The tobacco industry is constantly calling for more research into the links between tobacco and cancer. By calling for more research the tobacco industry is able to make itself look good - and at the same time to suggest that there is still some controversy and doubt about the links between tobacco and cancer.

But we don't need more research into tobacco and cancer. Everything we need to know can be summed up in four words: 'Smoking tobacco causes cancer.' And all we need now is a proper programme to persuade people not to smoke. But governments continue to spend millions fighting an unwinnable 'drugs war' against the users of cannabis, cocaine and heroin while they subsidise tobacco - a much more dangerous drug.

The tobacco industry isn't the only industry trying to cause confusion and doubt. Every cancer producing industry follows the same route: campaigning for more and more research and claiming that it is research and not prevention which will lead to a solution.

Consumers look on, puzzled and bemused. They quite like the idea of someone finding a 'cure' for cancer because it means that they can carry on eating the fatty food they like and smoking the cigarettes they enjoy without having to worry. 'Had such campaigns been at work during the Irish potato famine, which killed more than a million Irish between 1845 and 1849, they might have engendered studies into the biomechanical processes of famine rather than the social forces that gave rise to it,' wrote Robert N Proctor in 'The Sciences'. 'Investigators would have secured funding for research into why starvation ran in families instead of examining the social Darwinist policies of the Manchester era or studying how Ireland was able to export grain even during the worst years of the famine.'

In 1977 I estimated that the annual total expenditure on cancer research was probably close to $1,500,000,000. Today the annual total expenditure on cancer research is so vast as to be immeasurable. The National Cancer Institute, in the United States of America, has, by itself, spent more than $29,000,000,000 on cancer research! There are very few industries in the world which have grown as rapidly as the cancer industry - the charities, laboratories, research scientists and administrators who are devoted to the search for a cure for cancer.

The real irony in all this is the fact that money really isn't the key issue. You cannot 'buy' successful research. Although the huge cancer industry has spent a vast portion of its massive budget on laboratory research designed to find a 'magic' cure for cancer the majority of the most important and dramatic discoveries about cancer have been made by observant practitioners who have devoted themselves to a study of human patients and their habits.

In 'Paper Doctors' I explained: 'One of the most important breakthroughs in cancer research of recent years was made, not by researchers in expensive institutes but by a practising British surgeon, Denis Burkitt, working in Uganda. His first research grant from Government funds totalled £15 and his second, for £150, came from the Medical Research Council and was spent on an old jeep. By logical, patient study Burkitt managed to map the occurrence of a tumour common in children in that part of the world. He matched the map he prepared with other factors and eventually managed to show that the cancer was probably caused by a virus. Eventually he learnt how to cure the tumour. So, one of the most important discoveries was made, not by a professional researcher but by an observant doctor happy to continue his studies in his own time and at his own expense. Too many doctors these days are unwilling to begin any research programme unless they are first financed by an official agency and properly recognised as bona fide research workers.'

CHAPTER FIVE
LOSING THE WAR

The cancer industry uses statistics to try to persuade us that their billions of dollars are well spent. But I believe that if you look at the statistics objectively and carefully they show exactly the opposite. Although there have been a few (very well publicised) steps forward against some individual (and usually relatively rare) forms of cancer the overall effect has been negligible. I have absolutely no doubt at all that if the money spent on cancer research had been spent on teaching people what we know about the causes of cancer millions of lives would have been saved.

We are not winning the war against cancer. The war against cancer has been as badly fought as the war against 'drugs'. And it has been as unsuccessful.

Despite all the publicity and the extravagant claims the war against cancer (officially declared by President Richard Nixon in 1971) has been a failure. In the spring of 1995 the journal 'The Sciences' reported that: 'Five year survival rates for the majority of cancers (lung, colon, breast and stomach cancers, for example) remain essentially what they were twenty years ago.'

Leading American physicians and scientists have described the war against cancer as 'a medical Vietnam' and (rather more colourfully) 'a bunch of shit'.

In 1977, when my book 'Paper Doctors' was published I reported that 130,000 people died each year from cancer in England and Wales. By 1986 the figure had reached 140,000. The latest official figures from the government show that the figure has been going up steadily since then - it is now around 142,000.

'There have been some very important advances in cancer treatment over the last three decades,' said Dr John Bailar, who had been a researcher at the National Cancer Institute in the United States of America and had been, for years, editor in chief of the 'Journal of the National Cancer Institute'. 'But with respect to the cure of cancer, they are limited largely to the cancers that tend to occur in children and young adults, and those make up only perhaps one or two per cent of the total cancer burden.'

'Cancer deaths rates continue to go up year after year,' said Dr Bailar. 'Now these are real increases. I've taken out the effect of the changing size of the population, the changing age structure, declining mortality from other disease and we look at what's left. There is a genuine increase in the frequency of deaths from cancer, and this has been going on quite steadily for a number of years now.'

'Unfortunately, we have only managed to impact on the more rare malignancies with little effect on the most common and deadly forms of cancer,' says Dr Neal D Barnard in his book 'The Power of Your Plate'.

The cancer industry deliberately draws attention to its modest successes in the treatment of a few, relatively uncommon childhood cancers (putting pictures of children whose lives have been saved onto promotional leaflets and posters is a sure-fire way to keep the money pouring in). But there has been little or no improvement in the death rates for the big killers: lung cancer, breast cancer, prostate cancer or cancer of the colon.

None of this explains why governments have also failed to teach their citizens the facts about cancer. However, there are, I believe, two explanations for this seemingly mysterious state of affairs. Firstly, governments are always wary of annoying big, powerful, tax paying industries and there is absolutely no doubt that many huge, international corporations would be (to put it mildly) exceedingly upset if millions of potential consumers were warned of the dangers of smoking, eating or drinking exceedingly profitable substances. Secondly, (and I offer no excuse for the fact that this sounds extremely cynical) governments do not want people to live longer. On the contrary, they have a vested interest in people not living too long. People who live on into their sixties, seventies and eighties have to be given pensions and cost governments a great deal of money.

If you find all this difficult to accept just remember that although it is widely and generally accepted that thirty per cent of cancers are caused by tobacco, governments and Europe still subsidise the growing of tobacco. Governments spend a tiny amount of money trying to persuade their citizens not to smoke. But they spend one hundred times as much on helping the tobacco companies keep down the price of their products. It would, in health terms, be more sensible for these governments to subsidise the growing and distribution of cocaine. It is as crazy as if governments were giving muggers and bank robbers grants for the purchase of masks, guns and getaway cars.

'Americans worry a great deal about the import of cocaine and other drugs into the U.S.,' pointed out one observer sadly, 'but little is done to halt the far more deadly export of tobacco into the nations of the third world.'

Nor is it easy to explain why the medical profession has failed to teach people how to avoid cancer. Doctors have known the causes of most cancers for nearly two decades but very few indeed have done anything to help spread the word among their patients.

But the vast majority of doctors have for years earned their living by attending to the sick. Most doctors hardly, if ever, think about doing anything to keep their patients healthy. For example, I doubt if many people reading this book have ever discussed diet or nutrition with their doctors - even though a good, balanced diet is an essential prerequisite for good health.

Some doctors may make a little effort to persuade those patients who have already fallen ill to give up or cut down smoking but such efforts are usually superficial and rather uninspired. The trouble with doctors is, as I explained at some length in my book 'Betrayal of Trust', that the medical profession has been bought by the pharmaceutical industry. Doctors are educated by the drug industry and controlled by it and the result is that when the average doctor thinks of 'patients' he or she thinks of 'drugs'. Doctors are taught to respond to illness by prescribing a bottle or packet of pills. Many doctors (probably a large majority of doctors) have been so brainwashed by the powerful international drugs industry that they regard any treatment which does not involve drugs as hocus pocus and they regard preventive medicine as trivial, irrelevant nonsense which is rather beneath them.

Instead of putting energy and effort into teaching their patients which foods to avoid (and which to eat) doctors have created 'medical screening' - a high tech solution to a low tech problem.

The principle is a simple one: the patient goes to the doctor and the doctor (for a fee, of course) does tests which are designed to spot early signs of cancer or other diseases. But screening doesn't work. A once a year check up is no alternative to a healthier lifestyle.

In several earlier books I have explained why I neither approve of nor support the principle of medical screening programmes. But, as an example, consider, the much publicised cervical screening programme.

Cervical screening programmes have, over the years,consistently attracted huge budgets. Untold thousands of doctors have been employed in performing cervical smears. The laudable aim of the cervical screening programme is to reduce the number of women dying from cervical cancer and it is constantly being argued that if more money were put into cervical screening programmes thousands of lives could be saved.

But I don't think the evidence supports this contention. Indeed, a cynical observer might be inclined to suggest that it is the medical profession which has benefited most from the cervical screening programme. One leading physician described the results of screening for cervical cancer in Britain as 'disappointing'. A writer in one leading international journal argued that: 'there is no clear evidence that this screening is beneficial, and it may well be doing more harm than good'.

Although doctors around the world have strongly argued in favour of more expenditure on smears they have never really decided exactly which women need to be targeted. There have never been any trials done which show the undisputed value of the cervical screening programme. Amazingly, I don't believe that the cervical screening programme has ever been properly evaluated.

Indeed, the evidence rather firmly shows that cervical screening programmes may not be of any real value to women as a whole - though there will, of course, always be individual women who are able to say that their lives were 'saved'.

Statistically, the test has not been shown to save lives in any country where it has been introduced. Huge amounts of public money have been spent on organised cervical screening programmes but the incidence of cervical cancer has hardly altered in thirty years. In countries where the incidence of cervical cancer and the number of women dying from it are falling the rate of decline is no greater than it was before the screening programme began.

Britain, for example, has been spending over £150 million a year on its cervical screening programme since the early 1980s but the programme has never been based on any logical plan and the number of women dying from cervical cancer has hardly changed. In fact because the disease is relatively uncommon (cervical cancer does not make the top ten list of causes of death among women) huge numbers of women who do not have the disease have been subjected to unnecessary tests. Because 'false positives' are fairly common, many women are referred unnecessarily for further tests and treatment. Even more worryingly 'false negatives' occur in between 7 per cent and 60 per cent of smears. An enormous amount of anxiety and fear are produced by the often inefficient and thoughtless way in which smear reports are submitted to patients.

The failure of the screening test to save lives is not difficult to understand when you look at the available evidence.

The first major problem is that smear tests are neither accurate nor reliable. Different cytologists reading the same slide may produce entirely different results. Abnormal cells may be present in one sample and not in another from the same woman.

Most worrying is the fact that many of the smears taken by doctors are useless. One report concluded that ten per cent of all cervical smears sent to cytology departments were useless and a further forty per cent were of limited usefulness in detecting carcinoma of the cervix. The main problems are that doctors either take smears from the wrong site or use faulty techniques.

There is, surprisingly perhaps, still a considerable amount of confusion about the natural history of the cervical cancer.

From the evidence that is available it seems that some slow growing cancers do regress if left alone while fast growing cancers develop so rapidly that smears would have to be done every few months to be of real value.

One report concluded that a third of the biopsies performed because of positive cervical cytology are likely to have been performed for lesions which are insignificant or would have disappeared if left alone. Since biopsies are performed under anaesthetic (with which there is always a risk of death) it seems perfectly possible that the dangers associated with having a smear just may be greater than the possible advantages.

There is, not surprisingly, an enormous amount of confusion among gynaecologists about the best way to treat cervical cancer even when it has been identified.

Sadly, even when useful smears are taken the laboratories providing results cannot always cope. And even when laboratories do discover significant changes women are not always notified. Delays mean that at least one woman has died after having had a positive smear but before she had been given her results.

The enthusiasm of doctors for cervical screening is not difficult to understand. Sadly, I suspect that the medical profession's enthusiasm for cervical screening may, in part at least, have been aroused by and sustained by the profit to be made, rather than any belief that cervical screening will save lives. In one medical journal a writer pointed out that: 'unless doctors take urgent individual action a serious breakdown in cervical smear recalls - affecting GP income - could arise in five years' time.'

If the money spent on doctors' fees had been spent on educational programmes it is just possible that many thousands more lives could have been saved. For example, how many women know that it is vitally important that they should see their doctors straight away if they notice any intermenstrual bleeding, any bleeding after sex or any abnormal or unusual vaginal discharge?

PART TWO
WHAT IS YOUR CANCER RISK?

LIFESTYLE ASSESSMENT

Do this simple quiz to assess your cancer risk:

1. Do you smoke:
   - a) a lot
   - b) average
   - c) a little
   - d) not at all

2. How many hours a week do you spend in close proximity to people who smoke:
   - a) over 80 hours
   - b) 40 to 80 hours
   - c) 10 to 40 hours
   - d) less than 10 hours

3. Do you make an effort to cut your intake of fatty food?
   - a) yes - a big effort
   - b) yes - a small effort
   - c) no - not at all

4. Do you eat butter?
   - a) yes
   - b) no

5. Do you drink full fat milk?
   - a) yes
   - b) no

6. Do you eat full fat cheese?
   - a) yes
   - b) no

7. Do you eat red meat?
   - a) yes
   - b) no

8. Do you eat white meat?
   a) yes
   b) no

9. Do you eat fish?
   a) yes
   b) no

10. How much alcohol do you drink?
   a) more than one or two drinks a day
   b) one or two drinks a day
   c) less than one or two drinks a day

11. How much processed, packaged food do you eat:
   a) a lot
   b) hardly any/none at all

12. Do you eat smoked or barbecued food?
   a) yes
   b) no

13. Do you eat salt cured or salt pickled food?
   a) yes
   b) no

14. How much fibre do you think your diet contains?
   a) a lot
   b) an average amount
   c) not much

15. Does your diet regularly include citrus fruits (oranges, grape-fruit, lemons)?
   a) yes
   b) no

16. Do you regularly eat other fruits (eg apples, bananas, pine-apple, apricots, peaches, strawberries)?

a) yes
b) no

17. Does your diet regularly include cabbage, broccoli, cauli-flower or Brussels sprouts?
    a) yes
    b) no

18. Do you regularly eat garlic and/or onions?
    a) yes
    b) no

19. Does your diet regularly include whole grains (unrefined rice, wheat, oats, barley)?
    a) yes
    b) no

20. Does your diet regularly include potatoes?
    a) yes
    b) no

21. Does your diet regularly include carrots?
    a) yes
    b) no

22. Does your diet regularly include these vegetables: spinach, peas, beans, lentils, tomatoes, asparagus, kale?
    a) yes
    b) no

23. Are you noticeably overweight?
    a) yes
    b) no

24. Do you take care to restrict your exposure to sunlight?
    a) yes
    b) no

25. Do you take care to avoid spending too much time close to electricity wires and electrical appliances?
    a) yes
    b) no

26. Do you live near to a nuclear power station?
    a) yes
    b) no

27. Does your job put you in contact with any chemicals which might cause cancer?
    a) yes
    b) no

28. On average, do you have more than one X ray a year?
    a) yes
    b) no

29. Do you regularly take prescribed medicines?
    a) yes
    b) no

30. Do you regularly take medicines you buy yourself?
    a) yes
    b) no

Now check your score:

1. a) 50	b) 30	c) 10	d) 0
2. a) 3	b) 2	c) 1	d) 0
3. a) 0	b) 10	c) 20	
4. a) 2	b) 0		
5. a) 2	b) 0		
6. a) 2	b) 0		
7. a) 10	b) 0		
8. a) 2	b) 0		
9. a) 2	b) 0		

10. a) 5   b) 0   c) 0
11. a) 1   b) 0
12. a) 1   b) 0
13. a) 1   b) 0
14. a) 0   b) 5   c) 10
15. a) 0   b) 3
16. a) 0   b) 2
17. a) 0   b) 10
18. a) 0   b) 3
19. a) 0   b) 10
20. a) 0   b) 1
21. a) 0   b) 1
22. a) 0   b) 3
23. a) 7   b) 0
24. a) 0   b) 3
25. a) 0   b) 1
26. a) 1   b) 0
27. a) 4   b) 0
28. a) 5   b) 0
29. a) 3   b) 0
30. a) 1   b) 0

The higher your score the greater your risk of developing cancer.

 If you scored 100 or more then your cancer risk is danger-ously high

 If you scored between 75 and 99 your cancer risk is very high - well above average·

 If you scored between 50 and 74 your cancer risk is average.

 If you scored between 25 and 49 your cancer risk is below average.

 If you scored between 1 and 24 your cancer risk is con-siderably lower than average.

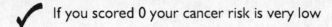 If you scored 0 your cancer risk is very low

If you want to reduce your cancer risk - read the remainder of this book!

PART THREE
FOOD AND CANCER

CHAPTER ONE
FOODS THAT CAUSE CANCER -
AN A to Z of EVIDENCE

You may be surprised to hear that there is now clear medical and scientific evidence available to show that nothing, not even tobacco, influences your chances of developing cancer as much as the food you choose to eat. It is estimated that between 30 per cent and 60 per cent of all cancers are caused by what you choose to eat. Doctors, scientists and supporters of the cancer industry claim that the battle against cancer will only be won with the aid of more money. They claim that in order to obtain the information we need we must spend, spend, spend. But that isn't true. It is not more knowledge we need (we have, as I pointed out in 'Paper Doctors' nearly twenty years ago, already amassed far more knowledge than we will ever use in our lifetime), but the ability and courage and determination to use the knowledge we already have.

Back in 1982 the National Research Council in the United States of America published a technical report entitled 'Diet, Nutrition and Cancer' which showed that diet was probably the single most important factor in the development of cancer, and that there was evidence linking cancers of the breast, colon and prostate to particular foods or types of food.

It is a scandal of astonishing proportions that a majority of the population still do not know about these vitally important and well established links. It is an even bigger scandal that a majority of the medical profession are unaware of these links too. Most doctors I have spoken to - even recently qualified ones - still dismiss the idea of a food/cancer link as mumbo-jumbo nonsense, preferring to rely entirely on prescription drugs, radiotherapy and surgery as 'treatments' for cancer. The average medical student probably spends more time staring down a microscope at histology slides than he or she spends studying the importance and significance of nutrition.

After he had seen a previous book of mine ('Food For Thought') advertised as containing material describing the

61

links between food and cancer one doctor sent me a very indignant letter, asking me whether I thought it was ethical to publish such statements as 'Between a third and a half of all cancers are caused by eating the wrong types of food' and 'You can dramatically reduce your chances of developing cancer of the breast, cancer of the prostate, cancer of the colon, cancer of the ovary or cancer of the uterus.'

(To be fair, after I had sent him details of a small amount of the evidence upon which I had based those statements, the doctor wrote back and apologised.)

I checked one large (over 1,000 pages) recently published medical textbook and found that the chapter on cancer summed up the role of food as a causal agent in just one, rather short sentence. I find this all extremely difficult to understand. I have been studying scientific research papers for over two decades and I have never seen such convincing research as that which shows the links between particular types of food and particular types of cancer.

It is not uncommon for new drugs to be launched after clinical trials which may have involved relatively small numbers of patients. In my book 'Betrayal of Trust' I pointed out that the number of patients studied in clinical trials before a drug is marketed is, on average, only 1,480 - and that the final, total, overall figure is sometimes much less than this.

In contrast some of the individual research projects which have been published showing links between food and cancer have involved tens of thousands of patients!

I have absolutely no doubt that if these undeniable links had been publicised by the responsible authorities (in medicine as elsewhere the phrase 'responsible authorities' is, I fear, oxymoronic) countless millions of lives and an enormous amount of agony and distress could - and would - have been avoided.

The suppression of this information by a greedy and conscience-free food industry, compliant revenue conscious politicians, a cancer industry dominated by grant hungry researchers and an uncaring, drug company dominated medical profession has, I sincerely believe, led to more deaths than any war in history.

Since the early 1980s the amount of evidence linking diet to cancer has grown steadily. In 1990 even the British Medical Association, hardly an organisation which would be widely described as revolutionary, supported the view that there is a link between food and cancer. Their published view was that 35 per cent of cancers, just over a third, were caused by the natural constituents of food and that another 1 per cent of cancers were caused by food additives.

Other organisations suggest that the link between food and cancer is even higher. The National Academy of Sciences in the United States, founded in 1863 by Act of Congress to serve as an official adviser to the US government in all matters of science and technology, has reported that researchers have estimated that almost 60 per cent of women's cancers and a little more than 40 per cent of men's cancers are related to nutritional factors.

Because I recognise that many readers may be sceptical about the claim that there is a strong link between diet and food (such scepticism will undoubtedly be enhanced by the fact that neither governments nor the medical profession have made much, if any, effort to publicise these links) I have in this chapter summarised just some of the scientific evidence which supports this claim.

My previous efforts to publicise the health values of eating a low fat, meatless diet have been consistently confronted by scepticism and opposition. It is my hope that this summary of just some of the most important available evidence supporting the contention that certain foods are a risk factor in the development of cancer will help settle this particular controversy permanently and may, perhaps, help other writers who may be tempted to tell their readers the truth about food and cancer.

I must emphasise that this list is not intended to be comprehensive. I have accumulated a list of several hundred scientific papers and journal articles dealing with the links between food and cancer (and many thousands more dealing with food and other disorders) and this list is merely intended to be representative - and to provide you with some idea of the breadth and importance of the available evidence.

If you would like to study even more evidence linking food to cancer (and many other diseases) then I heartily recommend the book 'Nutritional Influences on Illness: A sourcebook of clinical research', written by Melvyn R. Werbach MD and published by Thorsons. In a remarkably comprehensive and quite fascinating book Dr Werbach has listed and summarised thousands of clinical studies and scientific reports. He reports that: 'The cancers most closely associated with nutritional factors are breast and endometrial cancer in women, prostate cancer in men and gastrointestinal cancer', points out that 'the value of a low fat, high fibre diet in cancer prevention is well documented' and notes that 'avoidance of smoked, pickled and salt cured foods' has been shown...to be beneficial in preventing cancers of the gastrointestinal tract.'

Dr Werbach adds that 'there is early evidence that certain precancerous changes may be reversible with supplementation'. He reports that cervical dysplasia may possibly be reversed with folic acid supplements, that calcium supplements may help 'reduce the number of rapidly proliferating cells in the colonic epithelium in patients with family histories of colon cancer and elevated numbers of such cells compared to controls' and that 'vitamin A or beta-carotene reduce the percent of genetically damaged cells inside the cheek when betel quid, a tobacco like plant mixture is chewed regularly.'

Exhibit A:

Title: Calorie-Providing Nutrients and Risk of Breast Cancer

Authors: Paolo Toniolo (Epidemiology Unit, Istituto Nazionale per lo Studio e la Cura dei Tumori, Milan, Italy and Department of Environmental Medicine, New York University Medical Center, New York, USA), Elio Riboli (Unit of Analytical Epidemiology, International Agency for Research on Cancer, Lyon, France), Fulvia Protta (Pathology

Service, Ospedale Maggiore S. Giovanni, Turin, Italy), Martine Charrel (Unit of Analytical Epidemiology,International Agency for Research on Cancer, Lyon,France), Alberto M Cappa (Pathology Service, Ospedale Maggiore S.Giovanni, Turin, Italy)

Source: Journal of the National Cancer Institute

Date: February 15th 1989

Report: This study, which was conducted in the province of Vercelli in northwestern Italy where there is a moderately high incidence of breast cancer, was designed to investigate the role of diet in breast cancer and 'to test the primary hypothesis that fat and proteins from animal sources are associated with increased risk of breast cancer.'

The researchers questioned 250 women with breast cancer and a random sample of 499 women from the general population, using a structured questionnaire to identify the types and quantities of food each woman consumed.

After reporting that they had 'found evidence that the intake of total fat, saturated fat or proteins of animal origin is positively associated with the risk of breast cancer in women' the researchers reported that their 'findings had suggested that during adult life a reduction in total fat to less than 30 per cent of calorie intake, of saturated fat to less than 10 per cent of calorie intake and of animal proteins to less than six per cent may lead to a substantial reduction in the incidence of breast cancer in population subgroups with high intake of saturated fat and animal proteins in agreement with some dietary recommendations that have been made.'

'These data,' said the researchers, 'suggest that during adult life a reduction in dietary intake of fat and proteins of animal origin may contribute to a substantial reduction in the incidence of breast cancer in population subgroups with high intake of animal products.'

Exhibit B

Title: Dietary Habits and Prognostic Factors in Breast Cancer

Authors: Lars-Erik Holm (Department of Cancer Preven-
tion, Karolinska Hospital, Stockholm, Sweden), Eva
Callmer (Department of Medical Nutrition,
Huddinge Hospital, Huddinge, Sweden), Marie-
Louise Hjalmar (Department of General Oncology,
Danderyd Hospital, Danderyd, Sweden), Elizabet
Lidbrink (Department of General Oncology, South
Hospital, Stockholm, Sweden), Bo Nilsson (Depart
ment of Cancer Epidemiology, Karolinska Hos-
pital, Stockholm, Sweden, Lambert Skoog (Dep-
artment of Clinical Cytology, Karolinska Hospital,
Stockholm, Sweden).
Source: Journal of the National Cancer Institute
Date: August 16th 1989
Report: The link between dietary fat and breast tumours
was first described in 1942. Since then many other scientists
have published papers detailing this link in further detail.
'Dietary fat has been suggested as an etiological factor in human breast cancer because of the high correlation between
national per capita fat consumption and breast cancer incidence,' begin the authors of this paper whose study included
240 women who had surgery for breast cancer between the
years of 1983 and 1986 in Stockholm, Sweden. All the women
involved in this study were aged between 50 and 65 at the time
that their cancers were diagnosed. After analysing their results
the authors of this paper concluded: 'The results of this study
of mainly postmenopausal women and some premenopausal
women suggest that dietary habits have an impact on the prog-
nosis of breast cancer.'

'Study results indicate that dietary factors may act in breast
carcinogenesis,' continued the authors in their discussion of
their results. 'Several studies have found that these factors also
operate after diagnosis of the tumour, suggesting that dietary
habits are important even after a successful primary treatment.
The results of this study suggest that dietary patterns of the
western world (eg high fat intake and low consumption of carbohydrates and fiber) affect certain prognostic factors in breast

cancer, such as tumour size and ER (oestrogen receptor) content of the tumour.'

Exhibit C

Title: A Case-Control Study of Prostatic Cancer With Reference to Dietary Habits

Authors: Kenji Oishi, Kenichiro Okada, Osamu Yoshida, Hirohiko Yamabe, Yoshiyuki Ohno, Richard B Hayes and Fritz H. Schroeder; (these authors were from the Department of Urology, Kyoto University, Kyoto, Japan; Laboratory of Anatomic Pathology, Kyoto University Hospital, Japan; Department of Public Health, Medical School, Nagoya City University, Nagoya, Japan; Department of Urology, Faculty of Medicine, Erasmus University Rotterdam, The Netherlands.)

Source: The Prostate

Date: 1988

Report: In 1950 the incidence of prostatic cancer in Japan was about 0.4 per 100,000 male members of the population but by 1963 it had increased to 2.0 per 100,000 and by 1975 it was 2.5 per 100,000.

Observers have suggested that this increase (which is not unique, for increases in the incidence of cancer of the lung, cancer of the breast and cancer of the colon have also occurred in recent years) may be linked to the westernization of Japanese eating habits. During recent years the consumption of fat, animal protein, eggs, dairy products and oil have all increased considerably in Japan.

This study was of sufferers from prostatic cancer from 1981 to 1984 and patients suffering from benign prostatic hypertrophy (non cancerous prostate enlargement) and was conducted to find the risk factors for prostatic cancer. 'Two well trained nutritionists and one urologist interviewed each subject at the time of hospital admission'.

The findings included: 'Low daily intake of beta-carotene ... were significantly correlated with prostatic cancer development.'

Exhibit D

Title: Relation of Meat, Fat and Fiber Intake To The Risk of Colon Cancer in a Prospective Study Among Women

Authors: Walter C. Willett M.D, Meir J.Stampfer M.D., Graham A. Colditz M.D., Bernard A. Rosner Ph.D., and Frank E. Speizer M.D. from the Channing Laboratory, Department of Medicine, Harvard Medical School and Brigham and Women's Hospital, the Department of Preventive Medicine, Harvard Medical School and the Departments of Epidemiology, Nutrition and Biostatistics at the Harvard School of Public Health, all in Boston in the United States of America.

Source: The New England Journal of Medicine

Date: December 13th 1990

Report: The authors of this paper began by pointing out that in Western countries cancer rates are up to ten times as high as they are in many Far Eastern and developing countries. For many years doctors and scientists have noted rapid increases in rates of colon cancer among men and women migrating from low risk areas to high risk areas and these observations have suggested that the large differences which exist may be due to environmental causes rather than genetic causes.

The authors pointed out that two general dietary hypotheses have evolved in recent decades: firstly, that dietary fat, particularly from animal sources, increases the risk of colon cancer and secondly, that the intake of fiber reduces the risk.

This study involved observing 88,751 women between the ages of 34 and 59 for six years. The women, none of whom had any history of cancer, inflammatory bowel disease or familial polyposis, completed a questionnaire about their eating habits in 1980. By the year 1986 a total of 150 cases of colon cancer had been noted.

The researchers concluded that 'animal fat was positively associated with the risk of colon cancer' but that 'no association was found for vegetable fat'. The researchers found that women who ate beef, pork or lamb as a main dish every day were more likely to develop cancer of the colon than were women who ate beef, pork or lamb as a main dish less than once a month. It was also found that processed meats and liver with also 'significantly associated with increased risk'.

'The ratio of the intake of red meat to the intake of chicken and fish was particularly strongly associated with an increased incidence of colon cancer,' concluded the researchers, who also noted that 'a low intake of fiber from fruits appeared to contribute to the risk of colon cancer, but this relation was not statistically independent of meat intake.'

'These prospective data provide evidence for the hypothesis that a high intake of animal fat increases the risk of colon cancer,' said the researchers, 'and they support existing recommendations to substitute fish and chicken for meats high in fat.'

Exhibit E

Title: Dietary Fat Consumption and Survival Among Women With Breast Cancer

Authors: David I. Gregorio, Department of Social and Preventive Medicine, State University of New York, Buffalo, New York, United States of America; Lawrence J.Emrich, Department of Biomathematics, Roswell Park Memorial Institute, Buffalo, New York, United States of America; Saxon Graham, Department of Social and Preventive Medicine, State University of New York, Buffalo, New York, United States of America; James R.Marshall, Department of Social and Preventive Medicine, State University of New York, Buffalo, New York, United States of America, and Takuma Nemoto, Department of Breast Surgery, Roswell Park Memorial Institute, Buffalo, New York, United States of America

Source: JNCI

Date: July 1985

Report: The researchers estimated monthly fat consumption for a total of 854 patients who completed dietary intake interviews when they were admitted to hospital and subsequently estimated that 24 per cent of the women consumed between 500 and 1,000 grams of fat a month, 42 per cent consumed between 1,001 and 1,500 grams of fat a month, 21 per cent consumed between 1,501 and 2,000 grams of fat a month and 11 per cent consumed between 2,001 and 3,000 grams of fat.

They reported their findings as follows: 'Consistent with our hypothesis, an effect of fat intake on survival time was reported in this study' and concluded that the 'estimated risk of death at any time increased 1.4 fold for every 1,000 gram in monthly fat intake'.

Exhibit F

Title: Dietary Factors and Breast Cancer Risk

Authors: Jay H. Lubin, Environmental Epidemiology Branch, National Cancer Institute, Bethesda, Maryland, U.S.A.; Patricia E. Burns, Cross Cancer Institute, Edmonton, Alberta, Canada; William J. Blot, Environmental Epidemiology Branch, National Cancer Institute, Bethesda, Maryland, U.S.A.; Regina G. Ziegler, Environmental Epidemiology Branch, National Cancer Institute, Bethesda, Maryland, U.S.A.; Alan W.Lees, Cross Cancer Institute, Edmonton, Alberta, Canada and Joseph F. Fraumeni, Jr., Environmental Epidemiology Branch, National Cancer Institute, Bethesda, Maryland, U.S.A.

Source: International Journal of Cancer

Date: 1981

Report: These researchers questioned 577 women aged between 30 and 80 (all of whom had breast cancer) and 826 disease free women about their eating habits. They found that women who ate beef, pork and sweet desserts were significantly more likely to develop breast cancer than women who did not. They also found that women who fried with butter or margarine, as opposed to vegetable oils, and who used butter at the table were also more likely to develop breast cancer.

Exhibit G

Title: Role of Life-style and Dietary Habits in Risk of Cancer among Seventh-Day Adventists

Author: Roland L. Phillips, Department of Biostatistics and Epidemiology, Loma Linda University School of Health, Loma Linda, California, U.S.A.

Source: Cancer Research

Date: November 1975

Report: Seventh-Day Adventists neither drink alcohol nor smoke, most avoid the use of coffee, tea, hot condiments and spices and about half eat a vegetarian diet which includes dairy produce and eggs. In his summary the author noted that existing data on cancer mortality in Seventh-Day Adventists showed death rates that were 50 per cent to 70 per cent of the rates within the general population for most of the cancer sites that are unrelated to smoking or drinking alcohol. The author's studies showed statistically significant links between the eating of beef, lamb or a combined group of highly saturated fat foods and the development of colon cancer. 'It is quite clear,' he wrote, 'that these results are supportive of the hypothesis that beef, meat and saturated fat or fat in general are etiologically related to colon cancer.' He went on to say that: 'Green leafy vegetables that are quite high in fiber are negatively associated.'

The author concluded:'Overall, the currently available evidence on cancer among Seventh-Day Adventists is consistent with the hypothesis that one or more components of the typical Adventist life style account for a large portion of their apparent reduced risk of the types of cancer which are unrelated to cigarette smoking and alcohol consumption. Aside from abstinence from smoking and drinking, the most distinctive feature of the typical Adventist life-style is a unique diet whose principal feature is lacto-ovo-vegetarianism.' The author then added that other researchers had shown that the typical lacto-ovo-vegetarian diet contained about 25% less fat and 50% more fibre than the average non-vegetarian diet.

Exhibit H

Title: Diet as an Etiological Factor in the Development
of Cancers of the Colon and Rectum

Author: Margaret A. Howell, National Cancer Institute,
National Institutes of Health, Bethesda, Maryland,
U.S.A.

Source: Journal of Chronic Diseases

Date: 1975

Report: The author concludes: 'The evidence suggests that
meat, particularly beef, is a food associated with the development of malignancies of the large bowel.'

Exhibit I

Title: Nutrient Intakes In Relation to Cancer Incidence
in Hawaii

Authors: L. N. Kolonel, J. H. Hankin, J. Lee, S.Y. Chu, A.M.Y.
Nomura and M. Ward Hinds - from the Epidemi-
ology Program, Cancer Center of Hawaii, University of Hawaii, Honolulu, Hawaii, U.S.A.

Source: British Journal of Cancer

Date: 1981

Report: For this study 4,657 adults from the five main
ethnic groups in Hawaii (Caucasians, Japanese, Chinese,
Hawaiians and Filipinos) were interviewed about their diets
between the years 1977 and 1979. The researchers reported
that: 'significant positive associations were found for six of the
cancer sites: breast cancer with fat (saturated, unsaturated,
animal and total) and protein (animal); corpus-uteri cancer with
the same components as breast cancer; prostate cancer with
fat (saturated, animal) and protein (animal, total), stomach
cancer with fat (fish only) and protein (fish only), lung cancer
with cholesterol and laryngeal cancer with cholesterol. The
researchers also found significant negative associations between
breast and corpus-uteri cancers and carbohydrate intake.

Exhibit J

Title: Environmental Factors of Cancer of the Colon and

Rectum

Authors: Ernest L. Wynder M.D., and Takao Shigematsu M.D., both from the Division of Environmental Cancerigenesis, Sloan Kettering Institute for Cancer Research, New York, U.S.A.

Source: Cancer

Date: September 1967

Report: The authors of this paper concluded: '...dietary factors appear to be associated with the etiology of cancer of the large bowel. The dietary pattern that may fit the distribution of cancer of the large bowel includes a high intake of fats. The effect of this pattern appears to be more marked for cancer of the colon than cancer of the rectum.' And they added: 'There is a statistically significant association of obesity to cancer of the large bowel from the cecum to the sigmoid colon in men.'

Exhibit K

Title: Epidemiological Correlations between Diet and ' Cancer Frequency

Author: Pelayo Correa, Louisiana State University Medical Center, New Orleans, Louisiana, U.S.A.

Source: Cancer Research

Date: September 1981

Report: The author stated that: 'Strong and consistent correlations are reported between death rates of cancers of the colon and breast and the per capita consumption of total fat and of nutrients derived from animal sources, especially beef, pork, eggs and milk. Similar but less consistent correlations have been reported with cancers of the prostate, ovary and endometrium.' The author also reported that: 'Negative correlations of colon cancer rates and vegetable consumption are reported...Epidemiological data are consistent with the hypothesis that excessive beef and low vegetable consumption are causally related to colon cancer.' The author explained the link between the foods linked to cancer and the development of cancer by stating that 'these food items probably do not have a direct carcinogenic role but rather provide a microenvironment

73

favourable to the actions of carcinogens.'

Exhibit L

Title: Food Consumption and Cancer of the Colon and
               Rectum in North-Eastern Italy

Authors: Ettore Bidoli, Epidemiology Unit, Aviano Cancer
               Center, Via Pedemontana Occ, Aviano, Italy; Silvia
               Franceschi, Epidemiology Unit, Aviano Cancer
               Center, Via Pedemontana Occ, Aviano, Italy and
               European Cancer Prevention Organisation, Epi-
               demiology and Cancer Working Group, Brussels,
               Belgium; Renata Talamini, Epidemiology Unit,
               Aviano Cancer Center, Via Pedemontana Occ,
               Aviano, Italy; Salvatore Barra, Epidemiology Unit,
               Aviano Cancer Center, Via Pedemontana Occ,
               Aviano, Italy; and Carlo La Vecchia, Mario Negri
               Institute for Pharmacological Research, Via Eiritrea,
               Milan, Italy and Institute of Social and Preventive
               Medicine, University of Lausanne, Lausanne,
               Switzerland

Source: International Journal of Cancer

Date: 1992

Report: The authors studied 123 patients with colon cancer, 125 patients with rectal cancer and 699 patients with no
cancer. They concluded: '...the present study gives support for
a protective effect associated with a fiber rich or vegetable
rich diet, while it indicates that frequent consumption of refined starchy foods, eggs and fat rich foods such as cheese and
red meat is a risk factor for colo-rectal cancer.' The authors
found that a high consumption of margarine 'exerted a significant protection against cancer of the colon' and that 'high consumption of carrots, spinach, whole grain bread and pasta' reduced the risk of rectal cancer.

Exhibit M

Title: Diet and Lung Cancer in California Seventh-Day
               Adventists

Authors: Gary E.Fraser, Center for Health Research, Lorna Linda University, Lorna Linda, California, U.S.A., W.Lawrence Beeson, Center for Health Research, Lorna Linda University, Lorna Linda, California, U.S.A. and Roland L.Phillips, Lorna Linda University, Lorna Linda, California, U.S.A.
Source: American Journal of Epidemiology
Date: 1991
Report: The authors reported that: 'fruit consumption was the dietary constituent that showed a strong, statistically significant protective association with lung cancer...'

Exhibit N

Title: Dietary Habits and Past Medical History as Related to Fatal Pancreas Cancer Risk Among Adventists
Authors: Paul K. Mills Ph.D., W.Lawrence Beeson, M.S.P.H., David E.Abbey Ph.D., Gary E. Fraser M.D.,Ph.D., and Roland L. Phillips M.D., DrPH, from the Department of Preventive Medicine, School of Medicine, Lorna Linda University, Lorna Linda, California, U.S.A.
Source: Cancer
Date: 1988
Report: The authors began by pointing out that the foods and/or nutrients which had been suggested to be associated with an increased risk of cancer of the prostate included 'total fat intake, eggs, animal protein, sugar, meat, coffee and butter' whereas the consumption of 'raw fruits and vegetables' had been 'consistently associated with decreased risk'. In this study the authors found that there was strong evidence that 'increasing consumption of vegetarian protein products, beans, lentils and peas as well as dried fruit' helped to protect against cancer of the pancreas.

Exhibit O

Title: Increasing use of soyfoods and their potential role in cancer prevention

Authors: Mark Messina Ph.D, Diet and Cancer Branch, Division of Cancer Prevention and Control, National Cancer Institute, Bethesda, U.S.A. Virginia, Messina PhD, RD., Washington, U.S.A.

Source: Journal American Diet Association

Date: July 1991

Report: Most of the soybeans produced are used as animal feed but evidence has been accumulating that soybeans can prevent cancer. The authors of this report state that: 'Soybeans contain, in relatively high concentrations, several compounds with demonstrated anticarcinogenic activity.'

Exhibit P

Title: Dietary Prevention of Breast Cancer

Authors: David P. Rose and Jeanne M. Connolly, Division of Nutrition and Endocrinology, American Health Foundation, Valhalla, New York, U.S.A.

Source: Med.Oncol & Tumour Pharmacother.

Date: 1990

Report: 'A review of the epidemiological and experimental data suggests that dietary modification does have a place in breast cancer prevention,' say the authors. 'Based on present evidence, a dietary approach to breast cancer prevention should include weight control, when indicated, a reduction in dietary fat intake to approximately 20 per cent of total fats, and an increase in fiber consumption to 25-30 grams a day.'

Exhibit Q

Title: Shift From a Mixed Diet to a Lactovegetarian Diet: Influence on Some Cancer-Associated Intestinal Bacterial Enzyme Activities

Authors: Gunnar K. Johansson, Ludmila Ottova and Jan-Ake Gustafsson (the authors are affiliated with the Department of Medical Nutrution, Karolinska Institute, Huddinge University Hospital, Huddinge, Sweden).

Source: Nutr. Cancer

Date: 1990

Report: The authors of this paper conclude: '...the results in this paper indicate that a change from a mixed diet to a lactovegetarian diet leads to a decrease in certain enzyme activities proposed to be risk factors for colon cancer.'

Exhibit R

Title: Nutritional Approach to Oesophageal Cancer in Scotland

Author: Valda M Craddock, M.R.C. Toxicology Unit, Carshalton, Surrey, U.K.

Source: The Lancet

Date: 24th January 1987

Report: This publication took the form of a letter. The author began by pointing out that oesophageal cancer has a sharply defined geographical distribution in Britain - with many sufferers being in the north-west of Scotland where the consumption of green vegetables is believed to be low. The author also pointed out that oesophageal cancer is also very common in areas of China, in Iran, around the Caspian Sea and in parts of South Africa and adds that in all these regions the diet is low in fresh fruit and green vegetables - and the micronutrients they contain. 'A consistent finding from studies around the world of diet in relation to cancer is that consumption of fresh green vegetables is negatively associated with cancer,' writes the author. 'Deaths in women from this exceptionally distressing malignant disease total around 2,000 per year. Early diagnosis is not yet possible and treatment is unsatisfactory. Prevention, however, may be relatively easy.' The author also adds that the incidence of oesophageal cancer in Britain has almost doubled since 1970 and that 'there are epidemiological and experimental grounds for intervention studies which might lead to effective preventive measures, but nothing is being done.'

Exhibit S

Title: Cohort Study of Diet, Lifestyle and Prostate Cancer in Adventist Men

Authors: Paul K. Mills, Ph.D, MPH; W. Lawrence Beeson, MSPH; Roland L.Phillips, M.D. DrPH, and Gary E.Fraser M.D., Ph.D; from the Department of Preventive Medicine, Lorna Linda University School of Medicine, Lorna Linda, California, U.S.A.

Source: Cancer

Date: 1989

Report: For this study the authors evaluated dietary and lifestyle characteristics of approximately 14,000 Seventh-Day Adventist men. The men completed a detailed lifestyle questionnaire in 1976 and were monitored for cancer incidence until the end of1982. The authors concluded that: 'increasing consumption of beans, lentils and peas, tomatoes, raisin, dates and other dried fruit were all associated with significantly decreased prostate cancer risk.'

Exhibit T

Title: A Prospective Study of Dietary Fat and Risk of Prostate Cancer

Authors: Edward Giovannucci, Channing Laboratory, Department of Medicine,Harvard Medical School and Brigham and Women's Hospital, Boston, Mass, U.S.A.; Eric B. Rimm,Department of Epidemiology, Harvard School of Public Health, Boston, U.S.A.; Graham A. Colditz, Channing Laboratory, Department of Medicine, Harvard Medical School and Brigham and Women's Hospital, Department of Epidemiology, Harvard School of Public Health, Boston, U.S.A.; Meir J. Stampfer, Channing Laboratory, Department of Medicine, Harvard Medical School and Brigham and Women's Hospital, Department of Epidemiology, Harvard School of Public Health, Boston, U.S.A.; Alberto Ascherio, Depart ment of Nutrition, Harvard School of Public Health,

Boston, U.S.A.; Chris C. Chute, Department of
Health Sciences Research, Mayo Medical School,
Rochester, Minn., U.S.A.; Walter C. Willett,
Channing Laboratory, Department of Medicine,
Harvard Medical School and Brigham and Wom-
en's Hospital, Department of Epidemiology and
Department of Nutrition, Harvard School of Pub-
lic Health, Boston, U.S.A.

Source: Journal of the National Cancer Institute

Date: October 6th 1993

Report: The authors pointed out that: 'The strong correlation between national consumption of fat and national
rate of mortality from prostate cancer has raised the hypothesis that dietary fat increases the risk of this malignancy.'
By studying information relating to 51,529 American men
between the ages of 40 and 75 and sending follow up ques-
tionnaires to the men in 1988 and 1990 they examined the
relationship of fat consumption to the incidence of advanced
prostate cancer and to the total incidence of prostate cancer.

The authors found that 'total fat consumption was directly related to risk of advanced prostate cancer' and that
'this association was due primarily to animal fat ... but not
vegetable fat. Red meat represented the food group with
the strongest positive association with advanced cancer.'

The authors concluded that :'The results support the
hypothesis that animal fat, especially fat from red meat, is
associated with an elevated risk of advanced prostate cancer.' They also noted that: 'These findings support recommendations to lower intake of meat to reduce the risk of
prostate cancer.'

Exhibit U

Title: Risk of death from cancer and ischaemic heart
disease in meat and non-meat eaters.

Authors: Margaret Thorogood, senior research fellow, Department of Public Health and Policy, London
School of Hygiene and Tropical Medicine, London,

UK; Jim Mann, professor, Department of Human Nutrition, University of Otago, Dunedin, New Zealand; Paul Appleby, research officer, Department of Public Health and Primary Care, University of Oxford, Oxford, U.K.; Klim McPherson, professor, Department of Public Health and Policy, London School of Hygiene and Tropical Medicine, London, U.K.

Source: British Medical Journal

Date: 25th June 1994

Report: The aim of this research was to investigate the health consequences of a vegetarian diet by examining the twelve year mortality of vegetarians and meat eaters. The researchers reported: 'These data confirm the findings of previous studies that have shown a reduction in all cause, cancer and cardiovascular mortality among people who do not eat meat.'

The researchers showed a 'roughly 40 per cent reduction in mortality from cancer in vegetarians and fish eaters compared with meat eaters' and also added that 'the fact that total mortality was about 20 per cent lower in the non-meat eating group than the meat eaters is perhaps of greatest clinical importance.'

Exhibit V

Title: Risk Factors for Renal-Cell Cancer in Shanghai, China

Authors: Joseph K. McLaughlin, National Cancer Institute, Division of Cancer Etiology, Epidemiology and Biostatistics Program, Bethesda, MD, U.S.A; Yu-Tang Gao, Shanghai Cancer Institute, Department of Epidemiology, Shanghai, People's Republic of China; Ru-Nie Gao, Shanghai Cancer Institute, Department of Epidemiology, Shanghai, People's Republic of China; Wei Zheng, National Cancer Institute, Division of Cancer Etiology, Epidemiology and Biostatistics Program, Bethesda, MD, U.S.A; Bu-Tian Ji, Shanghai Cancer Institute, Department of

Epidemiology, Shanghai, People's Republic of China; William J.Blot, National Cancer Institute, Division of Cancer Etiology, Epidemiology and Biostatistics Program, Bethesda, MD, U.S.A; and Joseph F. Fraumeni Jr, National Cancer Institute, Division of Cancer Etiology, Epidemiology and Biostatistics Program, Bethesda, MD, U.S.A;

Source: International Journal of Cancer

Date: 1992

Report: The authors studied 154 patients with renal cell cancer and 157 controls. They reported: 'Elevated risks were observed for cigarette smoking...and for increasing categories of body weight and meat consumption, while reduced risks were seen for increasing categories of fruit and vegetable intake. An increase was also observed for regular use of phenacetin containing analgesics.' The authors also noted that these findings were 'consistent with earlier studies in Western countries and indicate that many of the same etiologic factors for renal cell cancer operate in low and high risk societies.'

Exhibit W

Title: Shift from a mixed to a lactovegetarian diet: influence on acid lipids in fecal water - a potential risk factor for colon cancer

Authors: Ulrika Geltner Allinger, Gunnar K.Johansson, Jan-Ake Gustafsson and Joseph J.Rafter; from the Department of Medical Nutrition, Karolinska Institute, Huddinge University Hospital, Huddinge, Sweden

Source: The American Journal of Clinical Nutrition

Date: 1989

Report: The authors concluded that: 'the consumption of a lactovegetarian diet may reduce certain risk factors of potential significance in colon carcinogenesis.'

Exhibit X

Title: NCI dietary guidelines: rationale

Authors: Ritva R.Butrum Ph.D., Carolyn K.Clifford Ph.D.,

and Elaine Lanza Ph.D from the Division of Cancer Prevention and Control, National Cancer Institute, National Institutes of Health, Bethesda, MD, U.S.A.

Source: The American Journal of Clinical Nutrition

Date: 1988

Report: The authors report that in 1986 it was estimated that 930,000 Americans would develop cancer and that 472,000 individuals would die of their cancer. The National Cancer Institute (the NCI), which aims to reduce cancer incidence, morbidity and mortality, 'believes that the potential for dietary changes to reduce the risk of cancer is considerable and that the existing scientific data provide evidence that is sufficiently consistent to warrant prudent interim dietary guidelines that will promote good health and reduce the risk of some types of cancer.'

The NCI suggests reducing fat intake, increasing fibre intake, including a variety of fruits and vegetables in the daily diet, avoiding obesity, consuming alcoholic beverages in moderation if at all and minimising the consumption of salt cured, salt pickled and smoked foods. The NCI believes that if these guidelines were followed there would be a 50 per cent reduction in cancer of the colon and rectum, a 25 per cent reduction in breast cancer and a 15 per cent reduction in cancers of the prostate, endometrium and gallbladder.

Exhibit Y

Title: Shifting from a Conventional Diet to an Uncooked Vegan Diet Reversibly Alters Fecal Hydrolytic Activities in Humans

Authors: Wen Hua Ling and Osmo Hanninen from the Department of Physiology, University of Kuopio, Kuopio, Finland

Source: Journal of Nutrition

Date: 1992

Report: The authors conclude that an 'uncooked extreme vegan diet causes a decrease in bacterial enzymes and certain toxic products that have been implicated in colon cancer risk.'

Exhibit Z

Title: Association between dietary changes and mortal ity rates: Israel 1949 to 1977; a trend-free regression model

Author: Aviva Palgi Ph.D., Instructor in Nutrition, Harvard Medical School, Nutrition/Metabolism Laboratory, New England Deaconess Hospital, United States of America

Source: The American Journal of Clinical Nutrition

Date: August 1981

Report: The author investigated the statistical effect of 'changes in food consumption of the Israeli population during 1949 to 1977 on concurrent mortality rates from cancer, heart disease, peptic ulcer, and diabetes mellitus'.

The author reported that: 'All the investigated mortality rates were in statistically significant positive association with increasing total fat consumption. Mortality rates of ischemic heart disease as well as of hypertensive and cerebrovascular disease were in positive association with both plant fat and animal fat. These findings suggest that reduced total fat intake may prove to reduce the investigated mortality rates.'

Note 1: Where I have included medical or scientific qualifications alongside the names of researchers it is because these were published on the scientific papers concerned. Where no qualifications are listed it is because no qualifications were listed on the journal articles I have quoted.

Note 2: In January 1986 the 'Journal of Occupational Medicine' published a paper entitled 'Cancer Mortality Among White Males in the Meat Industry'. The paper was written by Eric S.Johnson M.B., B.S.; H. R. Fischman D.V.M.; Genevieve M. Martanoski M.D.; and E. Diamond Ph.D. from the Department of Epidemiology, The Johns Hopkins University School of Hygiene and Public Health, Baltimore, United States of America. The authors studied 13,844 members of a meat cutter's union from July 1949 to December 1980 'to examine cancer occurrence in the meat industry'. They reported that a 'statistically significant proportional mortality ratio of 2.9 was obtained for Hodgkin's disease among abattoir workers' and that 'the results suggest that the excess risk of death from Hodgkin's disease in abattoir workers may be associated with the slaughtering activity'. They also found that meat packing plant workers were more likely to develop bone cancer, cancer of the buccal cavity and pharynx and lung cancer than workers in other industries.

I report this paper because although it does not show a direct link between cancer and the eating of meat as a food it does pose an important question: if human beings can get cancer merely by handling meat why on earth should there be any surprise that human beings can get cancer from eating meat? The authors of this paper also named viruses which naturally cause cancer in cattle and chickens and pointed out that these viruses are present not only in diseased but also in healthy cattle and chickens destined for human consumption. 'Evidence suggests that consumers of meat and unpasteurized milk may be exposed to these viruses. It would appear, therefore, that these viruses present a potentially serious public health problem.' Other researchers have made similar discoveries about a link between the meat industry and the development of cancer. A study of 300,000 adult white males in Washington State in the United States of America showed a 'statistically significant elevated risk of death from cancer of the buccal cavity and pharynx among butchers and meatcutters'.

CHAPTER TWO
FOODS TO AVOID -
AND FOODS TO EAT

However careful you are to avoid potentially cancerous chemicals cancer cells will occasionally develop inside your body. Most of the time those cancer cells are dealt with speedily and effectively by your body's defence systems. White blood cells find and destroy cancer cells in just the same way that they find and destroy bacteria.

Your body's natural immune system (and its ability to deal with cancer) will be damaged if you eat the wrong sort of foods - and will be aided and improved if you eat the right foods. Fatty foods will weaken your immune system and make your body less capable of fighting off those occasional cancer cells. When researchers studied the blood of human volunteers they found that a low fat diet greatly improved the activity of the body's natural killer cells.

Incidentally, it has been shown that as far as the body's immune system is concerned vegetable fats are just as bad as animal fats. You will protect your heart by reducing your animal fat consumption but in order to protect yourself against cancer you need to reduce your entire fat consumption - and that includes vegetable oils.

Vegetarians have more than double the cancer cell destroying capability of non-vegetarians. But this is not entirely due to the low fat content of a vegetarian diet. It is probably also due to the fact that vegetarians consume fewer toxic chemicals and no animal proteins.

And vegetarians have another advantage too: the ability of the human body's natural, killer cells to do their work is improved by substances such as beta-carotene which are found in considerable quantities in vegetables. (One survey of meat eaters showed that many could neither name nor describe a any green vegetables.)

Foods to avoid

✖ *Fatty foods in general*

The average diet still contains 40 per cent fat. Many official recommendations are still only encouraging a reduction in fat intake to around 30 per cent of the diet - despite evidence showing that a reduction to somewhere between 10 per cent and 20 per cent would make far more sense. Fat was the first dietary constituent to be linked with cancer and there is now probably more evidence damning fat than any other foodstuff. According to the National Academy of Sciences report 'Diet, Nutrition and Cancer' (published by the National Academy Press in Washington D.C., U.S.A. in 1982) there were at least six international studies published in the 1970s which showed a direct association between the amount of fat eaten and breast cancer incidence or mortality. In addition a state by state study published within the U.S. showed a significant direct correlation between fat intake and breast cancer mortality rates.

'Japanese women have the lowest breast cancer rate in the world,' says Dr Oliver Alabaster, Director of the Institute for Disease Prevention at the George Washington University Medical Center, quoted in 'The Power of your Plate', by Dr Neal D Barnard. 'Many Japanese women have migrated to Hawaii and the U.S. mainland. While marrying within their own community and keeping the population relatively unchanged genetically, they shifted their diet towards a more Western, higher fat diet and their breast cancer rate steadily climbed. A few decades ago the Japanese diet contained only around 10 per cent fat - today the average Japanese diet contains about 25 per cent fat. Within one generation it approximated that of Caucasian women living around them. This is very dramatic evidence that cancer is mainly environmentally induced, rather than genetically inherited.'

Peter Greenwald, Director of Cancer Prevention and Control of the National Cancer Institute in the United States of America also says that there is a great deal of evidence that fat increases cancer risk and points out that the differences in breast cancer rates in different countries cannot be due to other factors such as stress, pollution or industrialisation since there are highly industrialised countries such as Japan where stress and pollution are as high as the U.S.A. or Europe but where colon and breast cancer rates are low.

Since the mid 1970s there has been strong evidence to show a link between a high fat intake and prostate cancer. The National Academy of Sciences reports that an American study showed a correlation between a high fat intake and a high risk for prostate cancer. Studies in 41 countries have shown a high correlation between mortality from prostate cancer and intake of fats, milk and meats (especially beef). A ten year Japanese study involving 122,261 men aged 40 or older showed 'an inverse association between daily intake of green and yellow vegetables and mortality from prostate cancer'. Another study showed that vegetarian men were less likely to develop prostate cancer.

Other studies also confirm this link. In 1993 a study of 47,855 men, reported in the 'Medical Research Modernization Committee Report' revealed that those men who had high fat diets had a relative risk of 1.79 for advanced prostate cancer compared to those on a low fat diet. The investigators found that 'most animal fats were associated with advanced prostate cancer, but fats from vegetables, dairy products (except butter) and fish were not.'

The National Academy of Sciences reports that: 'other reproductive organs for which there have been associations between dietary fat and cancer include the testes, corpus uteri, and ovary'.

There is also a considerable amount of published evidence available to show that there is a firm association between dietary fat and gastrointestinal tract cancer. Some researchers have shown a link between dietary fat and cancer of the pancreas, and others have shown a link between fat and stomach cancer. Researchers have also accumulated strong evidence confirming a correlation between dietary fat and large bowel cancer (cancers of the colon and rectum).

The National Academy of Sciences reports that: 'In general, it is not possible to identify specific components of fat as being clearly responsible for the observed effects, although total fat and saturated fat have been associated most frequently.'

With all this evidence available directly from observations of human patients it is exceedingly difficult to see why such a large proportion of the cancer industry's budget is spent on performing experiments on animals.

Although the evidence showing that fat causes cancer is totally convincing (a United States Surgeon General has advised U.S. citizens that 'a comparison of populations indicates that death rates for cancers of the breast, colon and prostate are directly proportional to estimated dietary fat intakes') there is still a considerable amount of doubt about the mechanism whereby fat causes cancer.

One theory is that carcinogenic chemicals simply dissolve and accumulate in fatty tissues. If this is the case then people who eat animal fats will suffer twice for the chances are high that the fat they are eating already contains dissolved carcinogens. Another possibility is that fat may encourage the development of cancer by affecting the activity of sex hormones. Vegetarian and low fat diets reduce the levels of circulating female sex hormones such as oestradiol. Sex hormones are known to help promote the development of breast cancer and cancer of the reproductive organs (such as uterus and ovary in women and the prostate in men).

Despite the lack of clear evidence about exactly how fat causes cancer the final message is quite clear - to reduce your cancer risk you should make a real effort to cut back your fat intake - and that includes cutting out vegetable fats too. You should not make the mistake of assuming that you can avoid or cut down your fat intake noticeably by living on a diet of chicken and fish. Although it is widely believed that both fish and chicken are low in fat the truth is that even skinless white meat from a chicken is 23 per cent fat while most fish contain between 20 to 30 per cent fat and some are much higher - mackerel, for example, contains over 50 per cent fat. The only truly low fat diet is a diet which is mainly composed of vegetables, fruits, and whole grain cereals. Rice contains only about 1 per cent fat and no plant foods contain any cholesterol (although frying potatoes and turning them into chips can add a lot of fat!)

If you ignore this message then you are making a clear and conscious choice to accept a high cancer risk as the price for your high fat diet.

✖ Meat and animal products

Numerous researchers have linked protein with cancers of the breast, prostate, endometrium (lining of the uterus), colon and rectum, pancreas and kidney. And the type of protein which is most likely to cause cancer is protein obtained from meat.

The United States Surgeon General's Report 'Nutrition and Health' said: 'In one international correlational study, for example, a positive association was observed between total protein and animal protein and breast, colon, prostate, renal and endometrial cancers (Armstrong and Doll 1975). Similarly, a migrant study indicated an association between meat consumption and cancer of the breast and colon (Kolonel 1987).'

The Surgeon General also reported that: 'Studies have also found an association between breast cancer and meat intake (Lubin et al 1981) and an association of meat, especially beef, with large bowel cancer among Japanese (Haenszel et al 1973)...'

One possible reason for the meat-cancer link may be the fact that chemicals such as DDT tend to accumulate in animal tissues - and may be found in animal tissues years after their usage has been controlled or stopped. Whether it is the chemicals in animal protein which cause cancer is, however, a question of rather theoretical interest: the important point is that meat causes cancer.

There is evidence to show that Japanese women who eat meat daily have more than eight times the risk of breast cancer compared to poorer women who rarely consume meat.

There have also been several reports showing a high correlation between meat (an important source of dietary fat, especially saturated fat) and colon cancer. Beef has been specifically named as one type of meat associated with colon cancer. Several studies have shown a relationship between the incidence of prostate cancer and the consumption of animal protein.

Because most people who eat a lot of meat usually also eat a great deal of fat (because meat often contains a lot of fat) it is difficult to know whether these links between meat and cancer are a result of the protein in the meat or the fat in the meat. It is also possible that the link between meat and cancer is a result of mutagens being formed during the cooking of meat. And some experts have pointed out that carcinogenic fat soluble contaminants such as drugs and pesticides may be the reason why meat causes cancer.

However, I regard the question of how meat causes cancer as being of largely theoretical interest. The important thing is that most of us need to eat less protein in general - and since there is a link between meat and cancer it seems pretty clear that cutting out meat is a sensible way to cut down protein.

✗ Dairy products

The consumption of milk and other dairy products is relatively new in human history. And it is only in the 'highly developed' and 'westernised' world that milk drinking is considered essential or even normal.

Milk drinking (and the consumption of other dairy products) has developed because farmers and marketing experts have created the products and not because consuming these products is normal, essential or healthy. Babies need their mother's milk, taken direct from the breast, but no human beings need to drink dairy milk, or eat butter or cheese or other dairy products.

It is, almost certainly, the fat in dairy products which makes them particularly dangerous. Inevitably, therefore, some dairy products are more dangerous than others. Butter and cream and high fat cheeses are far more likely to cause problems than are low fat yoghurt, low fat cheese or skimmed milk.

But it isn't only the fat in dairy products which causes problems. There has for some years been accumulating evidence to suggest that dairy products can cause a wide variety of illnesses and there is now also some evidence to suggest that dairy products may be a contributory factor in the development of cancer of the ovary. The problem is, it seems, that a sugar in milk called lactose is broken down within the body to produce another sugar called galactose - which is then, in turn, broken down again. But if the consumption of dairy produce exceeds the body's ability to break down galactose this sugar may accumulate in the blood - and have an effect on the ovaries. Drinking low or non fat milk won't help this particular problem because the problem is caused by a sugar not fat.

✘ Alcohol

It has been known for some years that there is an association between alcohol abuse and cancer. In 1937, in France, it was noted that 95% of patients with oesophageal cancer were alcohol abusers. Another French study, published in the 1960s and involving 4,000 patients, showed a significant correlation between alcohol consumption and cancers of the tongue, hypopharynx and larynx. In 1964 the World Health Organisation concluded that: 'excessive consumption of alcoholic beverages was associated with cancer of the mouth, larynx and oesophagus'. A Finnish study, published in 1974, showed that chronic alcoholics were more likely to develop cancers of the pharynx, oesophagus and lung.

Alcohol has also been linked with cancer of the stomach and cancer of the pancreas. In 1988 the United States Surgeon General reported that: 'Reviews of experimental and epidemiological data suggest an association between alcohol consumption and human cancer that is strongest for certain head and neck cancers.'

Smoking seems to make matters even worse and there is a synergistic carcinogenic relationship between alcohol and smoking tobacco: people who drink a good deal of alcohol and smoke tobacco are particularly likely to suffer from cancer

Figure I

Dietary Components Which Cause Cancer

Selected Cancer Sites *	Fat	Weight	Alcohol	Smoked/Salted/Pickled foods
Lung			✓	
Breast	✓	✓	✓	
Colon	✓	✓		
Prostate	✓	✓		
Rectum	✓		✓	
Endometrium	✓	✓		
Oral Cavity			✓	
Stomach				✓
Kidney		✓		
Cervix		✓		
Thyroid		✓		
Oesophagus			✓	✓

* In descending order of incidence

The above table has been prepared with information provided by the United States Surgeon General of the mouth, larynx, oesophagus and respiratory tract.

You don't have to give up drinking alcohol completely in order to avoid or minimise this cancer risk. If you enjoy a glass of wine with a meal or a glass of whisky afterwards then that's fine. I myself am rather partial to a glass of malt whisky. But limit yourself to one or possibly two drinks a day at most.

✗ Food additives

Over 15,000 chemical substances are added to food as it is processed. Some of these chemicals are introduced deliberately (to add flavour, colour and consistency and so on) but many thousands of chemicals are added indirectly, either because they are used in food packaging or because they have been consumed by animals (as drugs or hormones) before finding their way into animal products.

Only a very small number of the substances added to foods have been tested for carcinogenicity and very few epidemiological studies have been conducted to find out whether or not there are any relationships between food additives and cancer incidence. At least one government has admitted that there are too many additives for them all to be fully tested. (The extent of the problem can be seen from the fact that any comprehensive testing programme would have to examine any possible synergistic activity between any combination of the many thousands of additives used).

✗ Smoked, salted and pickled foods

Substances which are potentially carcinogenic are produced in charred meat and fish because of changes in the proteins in those foods which occur when foods are cooked at very high temperatures.

Cooking foods over charcoal or smoking foods results in the food being covered with carcinogenic substances. In 1964 it was reported that beef grilled over a gas or charcoal fire contained polycyclic aromatic hydrocarbons (PAHs) produced from smoke generated by the dripping of fat from the meat onto the hot coals. Polycyclic aromatic hydrocarbons have also been found in a number of different types of smoked foods. Polycyclic aromatic hydrocarbons account for some of the potentially carcinogenic changes that occur in food during cooking.

The United States Surgeon General has reported that: 'International epidemiological evidence suggests that populations consuming diets high in salt-cured, salt-pickled, and smoked foods have a higher incidence of stomach and oesophageal cancers.'

The available evidence suggests that it is wisest to avoid food which has been salt-cured, salt-pickled, 'smoked' or cooked on a barbecue (see Fig 1 page 92)

Foods to eat
 *Fibre*
Until relatively recently fibre was regarded as an entirely inert substance - an unnecessary 'filler' that simply took up space in food, on the plate and in your stomach. There were even many experts who regarded fibre as a nuisance - something to be removed from food whenever possible. It was argued that because of its bulky presence fibre might interfere with the absorption of essential minerals.

The research work of Dr Denis Burkitt and other doctors changed that point of view for ever. It is now clear that fibre passes through the small intestines without being digested but that it removes harmful substances and helps to speed up the passage of food through the intestinal tract.

Once it had been recognised that people who ate a 'primitive diet' (rich in complex carbohydrates such as fibre) were less likely to suffer from a range of disorders, including bowel cancer, the popularity of fibre began to rise.

Burkitt noted that colorectal cancer (cancers of the colon and rectum) is rare among primitive people who eat unrefined foods.

Inevitably, perhaps, the food industry's immediate, knee-jerk response to this discovery was to start selling consumers bran and fibre supplements! Instead of encouraging people to buy more natural foods, full of natural fibre, the massive, international industry continued to sell packaged foods from which the fibre had been removed - but added a new range of foods which had been artificially enriched with fibre and many new varieties of fibre supplements. It was a trick of stupefying audacity, but it worked: all around the globe, in so called developed countries, people who regarded themselves as educated and intelligent consumers sought to balance their fibre deprived diets by purchasing and swallowing these artificial fibre supplements. Having paid the food industry to take the essential fibre out of their food they then paid the industry a second time to buy the fibre back.

Dietary fibre usually includes indigestible carbohydrates and carbohydrate like food components such as cellulose, lignin, hemicellulose, pentosans, gums and pectins - all of which provide bulk. The foods that usually provide fibre are vegetables, fruits and whole grain cereals.

Researchers are still trying to decide whether fibre helps prevent cancer directly or whether it works by helping to rid the body of carcinogenic substances. Fibre can dilute the carcinogens present in the large bowel; it can influence the composition and activity of the flora living in the intestine; it can affect the production of carcinogenic substances and it can speed up the rate at which food passes through the bowel (thereby reducing the amount of time that carcinogens are in contact with bowel tissue). Fibre seems to affect cholesterol metabolism and it also believed to reduce the levels of hormones which may lead to the development of cancer.

There is evidence that fibre helps to balance the cancer producing effect of fat in the diet. When you eat a fatty meal the gallbladder produces bile acids which flow into the intestine. The job of the bile acids is the help with the absorption of the fat in your meal. Bacteria which already exist within the intestine turn the bile acids into substances called secondary bile acids which are believed to promote the development of cancer. Fibre helps by having an effect on the bacteria in the intestine and, because it has a 'blotting paper' effect, by absorbing the bile acids. Because fibre takes up a lot of space it also dilutes the effect of the potentially harmful substances. In addition fibre is believed to delay the onset of menstruation in young girls. Girls who are brought up on a primitive, fibre rich diet start to menstruate several years later than girls who are brought up on a typical, fat rich, fibre poor 'western' diet. This is important because there is also evidence to show that the risk of breast cancer goes up as the onset of menstruation comes down. Just how fibre has all these effects is still the subject of some discussion although it has been suggested that specific components of fibre are more likely than fibre per se to be responsible for protecting humans against cancer.

As far as you and I are concerned, however, I believe that all this theory and all this research is only of academic value. The important thing to know is that your diet should contain a plentiful supply of natural fibre. You can get fibre from vegetables and beans and whole wheat bread, brown rice and cereals. Fibre is lost from refined grains and no foods made from dead animals contain fibre.

✓ Vegetables and fruit

One advantage of eating more vegetable products is undoubtedly the fact that by so doing you will inevitably eat few animal products - foodstuffs which are known to cause cancer. But fruit and vegetables have positive values too.

Vegetables and fruit also contain fibre - and some vegetables (cruciferous vegetables - cabbage, cauliflower, Brussels sprouts and broccoli) contain constituents (such as indoles and isothiocyanates) which are believed to have an anti-cancer effect.

A large number of scientific studies have shown that an individual's risk of developing cancer (particularly cancer of the gastro-intestinal tract - including the stomach and the large bowel) goes down if he eats more vegetables. No one really knows for certain why this is - but once again the exact mechanism by which the consumption of vegetables protects against the development of cancer is much less important than the existence of the relationship.

In 1972 it was found that the consumption of raw vegetables, including coleslaw and red cabbage seemed to protect against stomach cancer. In 1975 it was found that the consumption of fibre rich foods such as cabbage protected against colon cancer. In 1978 it was reported that individuals who frequently ate raw vegetables (especially cabbage, brussels sprouts and broccoli) were less likely to develop cancer of the colon.

Garlic and onions contain large quantities of a chemical which seems to have anti-cancer properties. People who eat large quantities of garlic and onions have less than half the risk of stomach cancer of people who either don't eat these vegetables at all or who eat them in very small quantities.

There are many other substances found in vegetables and fruits which seem to help prevent cancer. Phenols, flavones, protease inhibitors, glutathione and beta-sitosterol are just a few of the natural chemicals found in vegetables and fruits which seem to have an anti-cancer effect. And there is evidence to suggest that many vegetables and fruits contain antimutagens which help protect cells against the activity of mutagens -substances which damage a cell's DNA and can turn an ordinary cell into a cancerous cell.

There have been many attempts to explain the protective effects of vegetables but I believe the important thing is that the inverse relationship between these vegetables and the development of cancer (that is the fact that those who eat these vegetables are less likely to develop cancer) has been clearly and indisputably established.

In 1982 the American National Academy of Sciences concluded that there is sufficient epidemiological evidence to suggest that consumption of certain vegetables, especially carotene rich (i.e. dark green and deep yellow) vegetables and cruciferous vegetables (eg cabbage, broccoli, cauliflower and Brussels sprouts) is associated with a reduction in the incidence of cancer at several sites in humans.

✓ Whole grains

Whole grains (rice, oats, wheat, barley etc which have not been processed and had part of the 'goodness' removed) contain fibre, vitamin E and selenium - all of which can help reduce your risk of developing cancer.

✓ Vitamins and minerals

For the last two decades there has been a considerable amount of discussion about the value of vitamins (particularly vitamins A and C) in the prevention - and even treatment - of cancer. In vitamin A it is the beta-carotene content which is believed to have the protective quality. ('A large body of evidence suggests that foods high in vitamin A and carotenoids are protective against a variety of epithelial cancers', said the U.S. Surgeon General.)

Researchers have found that people who eat a diet which is low in vitamin A tend to be more likely to suffer from cancers of the lung, larynx, bladder, oesophagus, stomach, colon, rectum and prostate. However, vitamin A is itself potentially toxic and it seems clear that it is wisest to obtain your vitamin A as part of a healthy, natural diet rather than as a supplement.

With vitamin C researchers have found that this vitamin may lower the risk of cancer; in particular, it seems to lower the risk of cancer of the oesophagus and stomach. Once again it seems more satisfactory to obtain the vitamin C from a natural diet than from supplements. A diet which is based on or around vegetables and fruit will automatically contain a healthy quantity of vitamin C.

Despite all the billions of dollars worth of research which has been done no one yet knows how cancer develops. One theory is that free radicals - molecules produced routinely within the body - may damage the DNA within our cells, transforming a previously normal cell into a potentially cancerous cell.

Fortunately, it is now believed that there are some food substances called antioxidants which can neutralise free radicals which are formed. There are four known antioxidants at the moment: betacarotene (which is converted in the human body to vitamin A), vitamins C and E and the mineral selenium. Through their antioxidant properties - and their ability to neutralise free radicals these four substances are believed to be able to help prevent cancer (and, incidentally, to help prevent ageing and heart disease as well).

Because it can be toxic I don't recommend taking vitamin A supplements. But your body can get all the vitamin A it needs from vegetables and fruits. Foods which contain betacarotene include carrots, spinach, broccoli, apricots, asparagus, kale and peaches. Although some experts believe that vitamin C supplements are safe and helpful I prefer to obtain vitamin C from fruits and vegetables. Citrus fruits - such as oranges, grapefruit and lemons - are rich in vitamin C and many vegetables, including potatoes, broccoli, Brussels sprouts, cabbage, cauliflower, asparagus and tomatoes also contain the vitamin. Vitamin E is found in grains and vegetable oils and I personally do not think that supplements are necessary. Selenium, the mineral which is an antioxidant, is obtainable as a supplement but I don't recommend that you take it that way. Selenium can be toxic in large quantities (the U.S. Surgeon General has described selenium as 'among the most toxic essential elements'). You can get selenium in whole grains.

Your body will obtain all the anti-cancer vitamins and minerals it needs if you eat fresh dark green and yellow vegetables, fruits, beans and whole grain cereals.

Some of those who advocate meat eating claim that vegetarians are likely to have a diet which is deficient in iron. This is nonsense. A good, well balanced vegetarian diet will contain plenty of iron. Indeed, there is now evidence to suggest that too much iron in the blood (a problem which can occur among meat eaters) increases the chances of cancer developing. When iron has been absorbed the body stores it. In many westernised countries iron 'overload' is thought to be more common than iron deficiency. According to the American Physicians Committee for Responsible Medicine 'higher amounts of iron in the blood mean a higher cancer risk.' It also appears that

Figure 2

Dietary Components Which Prevent Cancer

Selected Cancer Sites *	Fibre	Fruits & Vegetables
Lung		✓
Breast		✓
Colon	✓	✓
Prostate		✓
Bladder		✓
Oral Cavity		✓
Stomach		✓
Cervix		✓

* In descending order of incidence

NOTE:
It is worth pointing out that a low fat, high fibre diet will also help prevent heart disease.

The above table has been prepared with information provided by the United States Surgeon General iron that comes from animal sources is more likely to cause heart disease.

Zinc is another mineral which is believed to have some beneficial effects on cancer risk. Dr Melvyn R. Werbach's excellent source book 'Nutritional Influences on Illness' lists three scientific papers which have shown that there may be a link between a low zinc intake and prostate cancer. One paper showed that serum levels in prostatic cancer are low when compared to patients who have benign prostatic hypertrophy. A second paper showed that prostatic tissue levels of zinc are low in prostatic cancer compared to normal men. And a third paper showed that prostatic tissue levels are low in prostatic cancer compared to patients with prostatic hyperplasia.

Sadly, there still seems to be insufficient evidence available for me to offer solid guidelines on the subject of zinc and prostate cancer. It seems a pity that the cancer industry (the recipient of billions of dollars in charitable contributions) has not done more work into this possible link. Prostate cancer is, of course, one of the major killers of men.

Zinc is present in rice, corn and oats, spinach, peas and potatoes and so a good, well balanced vegetarian diet should provide a plentiful supply. Since it is possible that too much zinc may cause damage I would recommend that you obtain your zinc from foods rather than from supplements.

Finally, it is worth pointing out that human experiments have shown that your body can repair the DNA which has been damaged by free radicals if it receives a plentiful supply of folic acid - one of the vitamin B complex of vitamins. Your body will receive the folic acid it needs if you eat a diet which is rich in dark green, leafy vegetables, fruits, dried peas, beans and wheat germ.

Foods which contain antioxidants
(beta carotene, vitamin C, vitamin E):

Apple
Broccoli
Brussels sprouts
Carrot
Cauliflower
Chick peas
Corn
Grapefruit
Orange
Pineapple
Brown rice
Soy beans
Spinach
Strawberries
Sweet Potato

✓ **Foods which contain folic acid**

Asparagus
Baked beans
Black beans
Black eyed peas
Broccoli
Brussels sprouts
Chick peas
Kidney beans
Lentils
Soya beans
Spinach

PART FOUR
OTHER CAUSES OF CANCER

CHAPTER ONE
DON'T SMOKE

There is a drug on sale in shops, supermarkets, airports, pubs and kiosks which has killed more people than the revolver, the machine gun, the hand grenade, the motor car, the aeroplane or the nuclear bomb. This drug has killed more people than cholera, smallpox, typhoid, tuberculosis, leprosy, malaria, yellow fever or bubonic plague. In the last half a century more than 45,000 scientific papers have been published proving without doubt that this drug, which is available without prescription, is responsible for a huge number of lethal or disabling diseases. The drug is, of course, tobacco.

Despite the publicity about the dangers of tobacco smoking and the protests from those who object to the pollution of the atmosphere the number of people smoking remains high.

In much of the developed world one in three adults still smokes and one third of teenagers are smoking by the age of nineteen. One reason for this is undoubtedly the skill with which the large tobacco companies plan their marketing campaigns and promote their products. For every ten people who give up smoking eight or nine non smokers take up the habit.

The cigarette is a perfect example of how science and industry have together turned a relatively harmless pastime (chewing tobacco leaves) into a dangerous addiction. Modern cigarettes are perfectly designed to ensure that the dangerous substances cigarettes contain are directed into the body quickly, repeatedly and conveniently. Tobacco is so powerful that just one of the 4,000 dangerous chemicals it contains is between 5 and 10 times as potent as cocaine. Tobacco is so addictive that only one quarter of the people who ever try it will ever succeed in breaking the habit.

There is enough nicotine in the average cigar to kill two people and the only reason why cigars and cigarettes are not instantly lethal is that the nicotine they contain is taken into the body fairly slowly. Nicotine has been reported to be six or eight times more addictive than alcohol and between five and ten times as potent as cocaine.

Apart from its poisonous qualities, nicotine has a number of undesirable effects on the human body. It stimulates the central nervous system and increases the electrical activity of the brain, lowers the skin temperature, causes blood vessels in the skin to become narrow, increases the blood pressure and the heart rate and numbs the taste buds. Cigarette smoke also contains several thousand other poisonous substances: for example, carbon monoxide gas. This reduces the oxygen carrying capacity of the blood and is one of the main reasons why heavy smokers so often complain of a shortness of breath.

Smokers are vulnerable to respiratory disorders such as asthma and bronchitis, to chest infections, sinus troubles, indigestion, gastritis and peptic ulcers. Many circulatory problems, raised blood pressure, arterial blockages and strokes are all known to be tobacco related. There is a strong link between smoking and heart disease - smokers are twice as likely to die of heart disease as are non smokers. Tobacco causes impotence in men and makes women infertile. When women who use it do get pregnant they give birth to small, sickly babies who are very likely to die while young. Children whose parents smoke are slow to develop - both physically and mentally - and are prone to more colds and chest infections than other children. Finally, there is lung cancer, the disease most commonly associated with cigarettes.

At the start of the twentieth century lung cancer killed no more than 10 men out of every 100,000. But just over half a century later 200 men out of every 100,000 were dying of lung cancer. Between 1954 and 1971 the number of male doctors who smoked cigarettes more or less halved - from 43 per cent to 21 per cent and the death rate from lung cancer among doctors fell by 25 per cent. But among the rest of the male population - who had not cut down their smoking - the incidence of lung cancer increased by 26 per cent. It isn't just lung cancer which is linked to tobacco. Other cancers associated with smoking cigarettes, pipes or cigars include cancers of the pancreas, the urinary tract and the mouth, larynx and oesophagus.

According to official statistics the majority of the thousands of people who have major surgery are smokers; 95 per cent of all patients with serious arterial disease of the legs are smokers and 20 per cent of the people who die of coronary artery disease do so because they smoke.

Despite all this well documented and well publicised evidence, and despite the printing of health warnings on all cigarette packs and cigarette advertisements, countless millions around the world continue to smoke. The vast majority smoke because they are addicted. Despite the fact that when smokers give up their habit they suffer clear withdrawal symptoms such as anxiety and restlessness there has, in the past, been a considerable amount of argument about whether or not people do get addicted to tobacco. It has, however, been shown that if smokers are given low nicotine cigarettes to replace their normal brand they will tend to smoke more of the low nicotine cigarettes. This evidence supports the theory that smokers can become addicted to tobacco.

Tobacco companies spend around $700 million a year on tobacco advertising in America and around $1 billion a year in Europe. If sponsorship and other promotional activities are included the total figure doubles. The alcohol industry is now the fastest growing sponsor of sporting events and tobacco companies have for years used sports sponsorship as a way of obtaining television coverage.

All around the world attempts are being made to introduce more and rules to control the advertising of tobacco but the big tobacco companies are powerful and are fighting hard - often with the backing of governments. For example, in 1991 the European Parliament voted for a total ban on tobacco advertising in all types of media but Britain opposed the ban.

The final absurdity is that although the European Community has, in recent years, spent a relatively small sum campaigning against smoking it has provided its tobacco growers with an annual subsidy of many hundreds of millions of pounds a year. It does seem obscenely hypocritical that countries which have spent huge amounts of money fighting the distribution and use of relatively harmless drugs such as cannabis should actually support the production of a far more dangerous substance which is directly responsible for millions of deaths.

Tobacco is the single most notable cause of cancer. In the United States of America cigarette smoking is reported to cause 400,000 deaths a year. If you do not smoke tobacco then your chances of developing lung cancer (one of the commonest types of cancer) will be dramatically reduced.

There is still some confusion and mystery about exactly how tobacco causes cancer (and the tobacco industry is still killing animals in its attempts to discover the truth about the link - a long running international research programme which enables the tobacco industry to maintain the myth that there is still some doubt about the existence of a link between tobacco and cancer and at the same time manage to convey the impression that the industry is anxious to find the truth). However, human epidemiological studies have provided all the evidence that could possibly ever be needed to prove the link between tobacco and cancer.

If you MUST smoke then the evidence shows that you can reduce your chances of developing cancer by eating plenty of fresh fruit and vegetables. In 'Food Choices of Health', the American Physicians Committee for Responsible Medicine points out that: 'A 55 year old male smoker whose diet is low in vitamin C has a one in four risk of dying of lung cancer in the next 25 years. But if the smoker has a high intake of vitamin C, either through diet or supplements, his risk drops to seven per cent.'

IF YOU WANT TO GIVE UP SMOKING
The first product sold to smokers wanting to give up the habit was, I believe, NO-TO-BAC which was marketed in the 1890s. Since then hundreds of companies and individuals have offered cures to smokers wanting help. However, it is my opinion that the smoker who really wants to give up can probably do so by himself without any professional aid.

Here is a technique for giving up smoking which I recommend:

Make a list of all the places where you smoke, putting the place where you smoke most at the top of your list and the place where you smoke least at the bottom of your list.

So, if you smoke most in the living room and smoke only rarely in the car then put the living room at the top of your list and the car at the bottom of your list.

Then give up smoking in each place in turn, starting at the bottom of the list and working your way up the list.

You mustn't go up your list until you can honestly and confidently claim that you've abandoned smoking at the lowest place on your list.

So, for example, your original list may look like this:

1. Living room
2. Office
3. Kitchen
4. Bedroom
5. Bathroom
6. Car

You should begin by giving up smoking in the car. You should only try to stop smoking in the bathroom when you never smoke in thr car. And so on.

The main advantage of this simple system is that you can give up smoking at an easy rate. And even if you can't give up altogether at least you'll have cut down your cigarette consumption - which will help.

Remember too that if you smoke because of stress and pressure you should keep the amount of stress in your life to a minimum and you should also learn how to relax your mind and your body.

Even if you have been a heavy smoker for years you will benefit in a number of ways if you succeed in cutting down: you will be healthier, you will live longer, you will save money, food will taste better, your teeth will be cleaner and your breath will taste sweeter.

As a bonus your family will be healthier too.

CHAPTER TWO
KEEP AWAY FROM SMOKERS

You don't have to smoke yourself to be killed by a cigarette. Tobacco is so dangerous that if you simply live with someone who uses it then your chances of developing lung cancer or having a heart attack are increased dramatically. At a world conference on lung health in Boston in 1990 it was estimated that passive smoking kills 50,000 Americans a year - two thirds of whom die of heart disease. That is, without a doubt, far, far more than the number of people who die from using all illegal drugs.

According to the World Health Organization tobacco smoke in the environment is responsible around one quarter of all the lung cancers which affect non smokers. A W.H.O. statement published in May 1991 warned that: 'in marriages where one partner smokes and the other does not, the risk of lung cancer to the non smoker is 20-50% higher'.

In America the United States Surgeon General claims that tobacco is responsible for around a third of a million deaths every year and the cost of cigarette smoking to America has been estimated at over $40 billion. In May 1991 the World Health Organization claimed: 'tobacco will cause about three million deaths a year throughout the world in the 1990s, including one million in the developing countries'.

Here is some of the scientific evidence which shows just how dangerous other people's exhaled tobacco smoke can be.

● In the UK as many as 1,000 non smokers die each year as a result of inhaling other people's cigarette smoke.
● Every year in the UK 17,000 children under the age of 5 are admitted to hospital because of tobacco smoke exhaled by their parents or people looking after them. The report, which reviewed 400 research papers, estimated that children whose parents smoke inhale the equivalent of 150 cigarettes a year. The same report also estimates that smoking by pregnant women causes 4,000 miscarriages of healthy babies each year.

• An American study concluded that women who breathe in other people's tobacco smoke are more likely to develop cervical cancer.

• Evidence presented at a scientific session of the American Heart Association showed that men who do not smoke are more likely to have heart disease if their partners do smoke.

• Researchers in London has shown that smoking in the home can stunt children's growth.

• British research concluded that breathing other people's tobacco smoke is a cause of lung cancer.

• An Australian judge has branded the tobacco industry guilty of misleading and deceptive advertising in claiming that there is no scientific proof that passive smoking was a health risk. After a 90 day hearing the judge, who reviewed evidence from the United States, Europe and Australia said the evidence showed that passive smoking caused respiratory diseases in young children, asthma and lung cancer.

• An American government agency concluded that passive smoking causes 3,800 lung cancer deaths each year in America.

• A U.S. scientist has estimated that passive smoking kills 50,000 Americans a year - two thirds of whom die of heart disease. He said that passive smoking ranks behind smoking and alcohol as the third leading preventable cause of death.

• Studies in America show that children of parents who smoke have an increased risk of heart disease.

The conclusion is simple: try to keep away from other people who are smoking tobacco. If travelling on public transport, eating in restaurants or attending theatres try to choose 'non smoking' areas whenever possible.

CHAPTER THREE
AVOID UNNECESSARY X RAYS

In 1895 a fifty year old Professor of Physics in Germany made an accidental discovery which was to have as great an effect on the practice of clinical medicine and practical surgery as any other single technological step forward in the history of healing. His discovery has also become the most significant cause of cancer among the various different types of radiation to which most of us are exposed.

Professor Wilhelm Konrad von Rontgen was an experimental physicist and in 1895 he was investigating the effects of cathode rays. What caught his attention was the fact that, although the tube he was working with was covered with black cardboard, a greenish glow seemed to come from a piece of paper coated with a substance called barium platinocyanide which happened to be lying on a nearby bench. Rontgen realised that the paper must have been made luminous by some unknown rays - something other than the cathode rays he had started off investigating.

Rontgen decided to investigate further. He put a thousand page textbook between the tube and his piece of coated paper and found that the paper still became luminous.

Next, he placed his hand between the tube and the piece of paper and saw the bones of his hands appear on the luminous paper as dark shadows. They were obviously dense enough to prevent the flow of these unseen rays - which had gone straight through the soft tissues of his hand. He had discovered X rays.

Doctors around the world soon saw the benefits to be obtained from Rontgen's discovery. At the end of February 1896, just under two months after Rontgen's original experiment, the British medical journal the 'Lancet' published a report from Liverpool which described how a surgeon had used X rays to help him localise an air-gun pellet before arranging for its removal. By enabling doctors to see inside the living human body X rays made it possible for physicians and surgeons to make much more accurate diagnoses than ever before.

Other research workers discovered that radioactive materials could be used to burn and destroy unwanted pieces of tissue. Doctors used X rays to make the hair fall out from the heads of children so that their ringworm could be treated more effectively. More importantly doctors found that radioactive materials could be used to attack cancerous growths. Pierre and Marie Curie were just two of the researchers who investigated the possibility of using radium as a therapeutic material in the early years of the twentieth century.

By the beginning of the twentieth century the risks associated with X rays had been well documented. A number of well known researchers died during the early part of the century. But despite all this evidence X rays were still used very widely. In the thirties and forties X rays were used extensively to look for signs of tuberculosis in the lungs. The result of this was that years later a number of women who had been exposed to these heavy doses of X rays developed breast cancer. By the 1950s it was clear that X rays could cause a great deal of damage. (Though, as a boy in the 1950s, I remember that shoe shops often contained a device with which parents and shoe fitters could look at a foot inside a shoe to see that there was room for the foot to move. Like many other children I delighted in looking at my feet through this publicly available X ray machine.)

By the 1970s doctors were beginning to worry that X rays might be killing more people than they were saving. Mammography (X rays of the breasts) had been introduced in the 1960s but doctors began to worry that mammography might be causing more cancer than it was detecting.

Doctors use X rays in two main ways: as screening tools and as diagnostic aids. These two techniques together make up by far the largest exposure of artificial radiation to which most people are exposed. The average dose of X ray used in a diagnostic X ray is estimated to be about as dangerous as smoking six cigarettes. Every X ray involves a risk and every unnecessary X ray involves an unnecessary risk.

In my book 'The Health Scandal' (first published in 1988)

I concluded that most X rays are entirely unnecessary. 'They are,' I wrote, 'potentially hazardous, they are extremely expensive and they are extremely unlikely to contribute anything to your doctor's knowledge of your illness.'

One of the first papers to have been published criticising the number of X rays done appeared in the British Medical Journal in the 1960s when a radiologist and a neurologist estimated that the consumption of X ray film was doubling every thirteen years. The authors concluded that their study gave 'ample evidence that the great majority of plain X ray films taken for such conditions as migraine and headache, did not contribute materially to the diagnosis.' They pointed out that much time and effort was wasted by doctors, radiographers and patients. Their plea for doctors to think before ordering X rays fell on deaf ears.

In the 1970s the British Medical Journal again printed an appeal for doctors to order fewer X ray pictures. By then it was estimated that the number of radiological examinations was increasing by ten per cent every year. This time the report in the BMJ pointed out that after routine chest X rays were taken of 521 patients under the age of twenty not one serious abnormality was detected.

By the 1980s the problem had become such an important one (and a global one) that the World Health Organization issued a statement saying that 'routine X ray examinations frequently are not worthwhile. Doctors,' said the W.H.O. 'ask for X rays as a comforting ritual.' The W.H.O. went on to point out that X rays are so overused and misused that they constitute a major source of population exposure to manmade ionizing radiation.

Today the situation continues to get worse. Many X rays are done because patients demand them ('Couldn't you just do an X ray to see what is causing the pain, doctor?' 'Wouldn't it be sensible to do an X ray to make sure that nothing is broken?'). Doctors comply with these demands because they know that if they don't, and something subsequently goes wrong, then there is a real risk that a court will find them negligent.

Taking an X ray just-in-case is now commonplace and these days most X rays are taken for legal rather than medical reasons.

CHAPTER FOUR
CONTROL YOUR WEIGHT

D o not allow yourself to become overweight. If you are already overweight then make a real effort to diet success-fully - and to maintain an acceptable weight for your height. Heart disease, strokes, diabetes, gallstones and some types of cancer are now all known to be made more likely by excess weight.

The United States Surgeon General, in the 1988 publica-tion entitled 'The Surgeon General's Report on Nutrition and Health', reported that: 'In international studies, a correlation between total per capita calories and cancers of the breast, colon, rectum, uterus and kidney has been reported (Armstrong and Doll 1975). Case control studies have found positive asso-ciations between energy intake and breast cancer (Miller et al 1978) and energy intake and colorectal cancer (Jain et al 1980; Lyon et al 1987). A positive association between increased body weight or body mass index and an increased risk for cancer has been observed for several cancers, including breast (de Waard and Baanders-van Halewijn 1974; Hirayama 1978; Mirra, Cole, and MacMahon 1971), kidney (Goodman, Morgenstern, and Wynder 1986), endometrium (La Vecchia et al 1984), and prostate (Snowdon, Phillips, and Choi 1984).'

One large study showed that the lowest overall cancer mortality was seen in men whose body weights were between 10 per cent below and 20 per cent above the average for their age and height. For women the lowest overall risk was seen in those whose weights ranged from 20 per cent below to 10 per cent above the average for their weight and height. Men who are more than 40 per cent overweight are 33 per cent more likely to die of cancer (with cancer of the colon, rectum and prostate the particular cancers they risk developing). Women who are more than 40 percent overweight are 55 per cent more likely to die of cancer - in particular, they are at risk of cancer of the breast, uterus (cervix and endometrium), ovary and gallbladder.

In the summer of 1995 a paper was published describing a

study of 115,000 female nurses in the United States of America. The women were followed for 16 years and the researchers found that one third of cancer deaths were due to excess weight. Cancers of the colon, breast and endometrium were all linked to excess weight. The study also showed that women who were obese were twice as likely to die of cancer and were four times as likely to die of heart disease as were women who were below average weight for their age. In a review of the study 'The New York Herald Tribune' reported that the results suggested that in the United States 'about 300,000 deaths a year are attributable to overweight.'

If you weigh just 22 pounds more than you did when you are 18 years old then you are probably at risk.

Use the height/weight tables opposite to find out how much you should weigh

Height/weight chart for women

Instructions

1. Weigh yourself with as few clothes as possible - and no shoes
2. Measure your height in bare or stockinged feet
3. You are overweight if your weight falls above your ideal weight band - your back will benefit if you lose weight

Height (feet & inches)	Ideal Weight Band (stones & pounds)
4.10	7.5 - 8.5
4.11	7.7 - 8.7
5.0	7.9 - 8.9
5.1	7.11 - 8.11
5.2	8.1 - 9.1
5.3	8.4 - 9.4
5.4	8.6 - 9.6
5.5	8.10 - 9.10
5.6	9.0 - 10.0
5.7	9.3 - 10.3
5.8	9.7 - 10.7
5.9	9.10 - 10.10
5.10	10.0 - 11.0
5.11	10.3 - 11.3
6.0	10.7 - 11.7
6.1	10.9 - 11.9
6.2	10.12-11.12
6.3	11.2 - 12.2
6.4	11.5 - 12.5
6.5	11.8 - 12.8
6.6	12.0 - 13.0

NOTE

Ideal weights vary with age and various other factors. But if you weigh more than 14 pounds above the maximum in your Ideal Weight Band then your weight will almost certainly be having an adverse effect on your health.

Height/weight chart for men

Instructions
1. Weigh yourself with as few clothes as possible - and no shoes
2. Measure your height in bare or stockinged feet
3. You are overweight if your weight falls above your ideal weight band - your back will benefit if you lose weight

Height (feet & inches)	Ideal Weight Band (stones & pounds)
5.0	8.5 - 9.5
5.1	8.6 - 9.6
5.2	8.7 - 9.7
5.3	8.8 - 9.8
5.4	8.11 - 9.11
5.5	9.2 - 10.2
5.6	9.6 - 10.6
5.7	9.10 - 10.10
5.8	10.0 - 11.0
5.9	10.4 - 11.4
5.10	10.8 - 11.8
5.11	10.12-11.12
6.0	11.2 - 12.2
6.1	11.6 - 12.6
6.2	11.10-12.10
6.3	12.0 - 13.0
6.4	12.4 - 13.4
6.5	12.8 - 13.8
6.6	13.0 - 14.0

NOTE

Ideal weights vary with age and various other factors. But if you weigh more than 14 pounds above the maximum in your Ideal Weight Band then your weight will almost certainly be having an adverse effect on your health.

CHAPTER FIVE
BEWARE OF SUNLIGHT

The link between sunlight and skin cancer was already established by the end of the nineteenth century. Every few years doctors do their best to frighten patients into spending less time in the sunshine - or covering up their skin when they are in the sun. But although these scares produce some behavioural changes in a few people the vast majority of citizens ignore the advice.

One young woman I know, a keen sunbed enthusiast, needed to have a small, possibly cancerous blemish removed from her arm. She continued to use a sunbed while waiting for the operation to have the possible skin cancer removed and she continued to spend several days a week keeping her skin brown after the possible skin cancer had been removed - even though the risks she was taking were explained to her at some length.

In my opinion most cases of skin cancer are optional. Unlike tobacco smokers and heavy drinkers suntan worshippers do not even have the excuse that their recklessness is inspired by an unbreakable physiological or psychological addiction.

CHAPTER SIX
AVOID FOOD ADDITIVES

On average, each one of us eats around 5.5lb (2.5kg) of additives every year. Food manufacturers use additives as flavourings, preservatives and colourings. They use them to improve the taste, shelf life and texture of the foods they sell.

In one booklet published by a government agency readers were told that 'ham and bacon couldn't be sold without the preservative that also gives them their pink colour'. The authors of the booklet claimed that 'scientists and doctors who check safety evidence for the government are satisfied the use of these additives is safe.'

In the same booklet the government agency admitted that flavourings are not controlled as tightly as other additives because there are over 3,000 of them in use, in many different combinations!

In no area of medicine is the difference between animals and human beings illustrated more vividly than in the study of food constituents and food additives. Many substances which occur naturally in plants are known to be carcinogenic if eaten by animals. If we refused to eat foods containing substances known to be carcinogenic to other species there would be very little indeed left for us to eat.

Food ingredients which may cause cancer in humans include the polycyclic aromatic hydrocarbons (the concentration of which is increased by burning, overcooking or barbecuing); the nitrosamines (which may be formed by a reaction between substances normally present in food and the nitrites or nitrates which are added to fish, sausages, bacon, ham, cheese etc in order to stop the food from 'spoiling') and moulds which grow on foods which are normally free of carcinogens and then produce toxic substances called mycotoxins (the fungus called ergot which grows on rye and causes womb contractions in healthy women has been used as a prescription drug and is the substance from which LSD was created). The aflatoxins, which grow on peanuts, are among the most powerful of all carcinogenic substances.

It is, however, the artificially additives which are added to food as preservatives, colourings and flavourings which worry consumers most. Theoretically, chemicals which are added to food are subjected to extensive testing to make sure that they are not dangerous. But the value of many of the tests which are performed must be in question. 'The interpretation of studies which appear to show the potential for tumour formation in animals is becoming increasing difficult,' said the British Medical Association in its book 'The BMA Guide to Living With Risk' (published by Penguin in 1990). 'Some testing procedures are very tightly standardised, but have little relationship to the real world or to use by humans. Other tests are more flexible but difficult to relate one to the other. Indeed, a great deal more needs to be known about the induction of cancer in animals by chemicals before the findings can be confidently related to man.' (One wonders why scientists don't just forget about the animal experiments completely and concentrate on human studies. They could do preliminary toxicity and carcinogenicity tests on human tissue and organ samples and then study limited cohort samples in order to investigate the long term carcinogenicity in humans).

'Chemicals that cause cancer are a diverse group which act in different ways,' says the British Medical Association. 'To classify all of them for the purpose of regulation as 'carcinogens' is not very logical today, because we really do not know what some of the laboratory findings in animals actually mean, and the mechanism of action of chemical carcinogens in biochemical terms is very unclear. Some of the testing defies common sense. If a chemical is administered to a rat in relatively enormous amounts there will be absolutely inevitable changes in that part of the diet which remains and is acceptable to that unfortunate animal, its metabolism is bound to be altered, and these changes may or may not have as much influence on the animal's illness as the chemical itself.'

'In summary, then,' said the B.M.A., 'carcinogens in

food are more likely to be there 'naturally' or as a result of traditional preservation methods than by the addition of synthetic chemicals. The significance to human beings of very tiny amounts of carcinogens (as assessed through animal experimentation) is unknown. It would be hard to live on a diet which contained no substances which at some time had been shown by laboratory or animal tests to have carcinogenic properties.'

The British Medical Association has also pointed out that: 'if salt and sugar were being tested as potential food additives today, and if judgement of acceptability was to be based purely on the laboratory and animal testing, it is unlikely that either would be permitted for use in food.'

In my view food additives are potential hazards. They are best avoided as much as possible and this is best done by eating as much fresh food as possible.

CHAPTER SEVEN:
THE DANGER OF ELECTRICITY

Electricity is almost certainly more dangerous than you think. If you spend most of your time working with or close to an electrical appliance, if you live or work near to an electricity supply line or if you spend your days working with electrical equipment then the chances of you developing cancer of one sort or another are considerably increased.

Of course, the men in empty suits won't tell you this. They'll frighten you half to death about minority threats such as AIDS and radon because the former is politically useful and the latter seems like an excellent way to boost the building industry but they won't give you any warning about the danger of electricity because they don't want to annoy the many large and powerful business interests which sell, market, service or supply electricity and electrical equipment.

But the evidence is pretty convincing; and in America, where people only vote with their wallets when they really believe something, house prices near to electricity supply lines have fallen by as much as a quarter.

Just look at these facts:

● The dean of a school of public health said: 'The present state of affairs is like the correlation between smoking and lung cancer 30 years ago'. He added that, at a conservative estimate, a third of all childhood cancers are caused by electrical fields.

● A study of nearly 500 children showed that children whose mothers used electric blankets when they were pregnant were two and a half times as likely to develop brain tumours.

● A study of nearly 700 children showed that children who lived in houses near to power distribution lines were two or three times as likely to die of leukaemia or brain tumours.

● A study at an American University showed that men who work as electricians or electrical engineers are ten times as likely to develop certain types of brain tumour.

● Experts found that workers for a telephone company who worked alongside electricity power lines were seven times as likely to develop leukaemia.

And so it goes on. The evidence is extremely convincing. In my view the only real task left is to quantify the risks accurately. And that is proving difficult. And, you may not be surprised to hear, it is taking time.

Meanwhile, what can you do to reduce your chances - and the chances of anyone in your family - of being killed by electrical fields?

✘ Don't have mains powered radios, answering machines, clocks or other electrical devices unnecessarily close to you - on your desk, in the kitchen or by your bed. Battery operated appliances are probably safer.

✘ Don't sit within two and a half or three feet of the front sides or the back of a Visual Display Terminal on a computer or word processor.

✘ If you are pregnant try to keep away from Visual DisplayTerminals completely. A study of over 1,500 women showed that pregnant women who spend more than 20 hours a week working on such terminals have a much greater chance of having a miscarriage.

✘ If your child's school is within 150 yards of a major electricity supply line ask the authorities to test the electrical fields in classrooms, playground and sports fields.

✘ Don't sit (and don't let children sit) closer than three feet from your television set when it is switched on. TV sets produce potentially dangerous electrical fields which are stronger the closer you get.

✘Unplug electrical blankets before you get into bed.

✘ Don't sit or stand in front of household appliances such as microwave ovens when they are switched on.

✘ Try not to live in a home within 150 yards of a major electricity supply line. I think this is probably particularly important if you have small children or are pregnant.

CHAPTER EIGHT
OCCUPATIONAL AND INDUSTRIAL CANCERS

Here is what I wrote about occupational cancers in my book 'Paper Doctors' back in 1977: 'In 1775 a prominent English surgeon, Percival Pott, described cancer of the scrotum in chimney sweeps. Since then many other occupational and environmental relationships have been found. It has been proved that wood can cause cancer of the nasopharynx and cancer of the sinuses, that tobacco causes cancer of the tongue, pharynx, lung and oesophagus, and that alcohol causes cancer of the oesophagus. Diets low in fresh vegetables and fruit are likely to result in cancer of the stomach. Occupational cancers are common these days because of new methods of manufacture, waste disposal, power production and food processing. Rubber workers are in danger of developing bladder cancer and workers exposed to cutting oil are particularly likely to develop skin cancers. Sadly, this list expands month by month.'

'The introduction of synthetic chemicals into such things as pesticides, agricultural preparations, food additives and cosmetics means that many millions of people may be exposed to harmful carcinogenic substances.'

I reported that experts had noted that 'over 70 per cent of human cancers are probably wholly or partly caused by chemicals' and that they had shown 'that despite the well-known historical association between soot and scrotal cancer, there are still cases of cancer caused by similar substances.'

I pointed out that one region alone had recorded 187 cases of scrotal cancer between 1950 and 1967 and that at least two-thirds of these men had worked with mineral oils. I also reported that mineral oil mists had been listed as causes of scrotal cancer among lathe workers.

'...there is now evidence that exposure to tar fumes is also linked with the development of cancer,' I wrote, pointing out that studies among gas workers had shown an increase in the incidence of lung cancer, cancer of the bladder, cancer of the skin and cancer of the scrotum. I added that an increase in the incidence of lung cancer has also been reported from doctors studying gas workers in North America.

'Workers in paint factories, textile factories, printing works and in work involving the use of tar, pitch and gas are at risk from other substances which have in recent years been shown to act as carcinogens,' I wrote. 'Workers in chemical, rubber and cable making industries are also listed as being at risk.' I quoted one publication estimating 'that in some industrial communities the incidence of occupational bladder cancers may be running at about 20 per cent.'

'The manufacturing processes used in the preparation of polyvinyl chloride (PVC) have been unchanged for several decades, but it was not until 1974 that it was shown that workers in the industry were developing liver cancer. Work done in the United States, Great Britain, Scandinavia, West Germany, France, Italy, Romania and Czechoslovakia has supported this observation. Workers involved in using asbestos have a greater chance of developing lung cancers, as do workers exposed to small amounts of arsenic,' I wrote.

Little has changed since all that was written nineteen years ago. Millions of workers around the world are still regularly exposed to cancer inducing chemicals. The evidence showing the existence of the links between chemicals and cancers is indisputable but no one seems to care or take any notice. Company directors and executives nod pseudosympathetically and call for yet more research to substantiate what is already known. Politicians, bribed either by the tax dollars those companies are contributing or by personal campaign contributions, turn a blind eye. Union officials either ignore the evidence or use it to obtain another 2 per cent pay rise. The workers whose lives are at risk put their faith in the abilities of the medical establishment and the pharmaceutical industry to find cures for the cancers they know they will get.

CHAPTER NINE
PESTICIDES

'For the first time in the history of the world every human being is subject to contact with dangerous chemicals from the moment of conception until death,' wrote Rachel Carson. The book she published in 1962, 'Silent Spring', drew attention to the deadly effects of pesticides such as DDT.

Today, little has changed - except that we spray and smother our world and our food with ever more pesticides. Chemicals are used to kill weeds, insects, bacteria, fungi and animals which threaten the production and profitability of crops.

Once again the safety - or danger - of these chemicals has been confused by the use of vast numbers of animal experiments. Many chemicals cause birth defects in laboratory animals but these chemicals are still put on the market and used widely on the grounds that animals are so different to human beings that the results of the experiments cannot be used to make any sort of useful judgement about what effect the chemical may have on human beings. And yet no other tests or studies are done! Scientists and politicians rely upon animal experiments which are so misleading that they are worthless.

Just how dangerous all these chemicals are is, therefore, a complete mystery. Some observers now believe that it is through the accumulation of these chemicals in fatty tissue that cancer is triggered. This makes complete sense to me and seems a logical explanation of the fact that a diet that contains too much fat and obesity are both linked to the development of many different types of cancer.

There is little you or I can do to reduce our exposure to pesticides or chemicals. But we can reduce the amount of fat we eat - and we can control our weight.

CHAPTER TEN
NUCLEAR POWER

Nuclear power is, without a doubt, the source of cancer- inducing radiation which most people worry about most. Studies have shown that children born in homes close to nuclear plants, or born to fathers who worked in nuclear plants, are more likely to suffer from diseases such as leukaemia. I believe that there is undoubtedly a cancer risk involved in the use of nuclear power but that this risk is significantly lower than the risks created by the overuse of X rays.

CHAPTER ELEVEN
RADON

In recent years the risk of radon gas has been given much publicity. Many people undoubtedly worry that they are being poisoned in their homes by radon gas. In Britain, the Government published thousands of special radon warning leaflets suggesting that thousands of people were at risk of being killed in the safety of their own homes.

The official leaflet explained that radon gas comes from the radioactive decay of uranium found in soil and rocks - and that it seeps into houses through cracks in the floors. The British Government claimed that if a home contained too much radon then the houseowner's chances of developing lung cancer might be increased dramatically.

The Government estimated that at least a quarter of a million people were being poisoned by radon - and that 1750 to 2500 people in the United Kingdom would develop lung cancer every year because of it.

But independent experts claimed that the radon scare the Government was starting was unjustified.

Homeowners whose houses, bungalows or flats contained too much radon were given immensely complicated instructions on how to stop the radon gas seeping into their homes and endangering their health.

Here are some of the instructions they received:

✗ Don't have open fires and block up your chimneys

✓ Leave downstairs windows partially open

✓ If your skirting boards are loose take them off and refix them

✓ Cover your floors with reinforced polythene to stop radon gas seeping through

✓ Cover the polythene with hardboard and nail it down (they don't seem worried about the gas seeping through the nail holes)

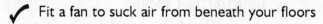

✓ Fit a fan to suck air from beneath your floors

✓ Dig out a pit underneath your house

Ironically, if radon had built up in British homes it was partly because of the Government's own policy of encouraging house-holders to draught proof and 'seal' their homes. Homeowners who followed the Government's last lot of advice - and fitted good draughtproofing and double glazing - were suddenly those most seriously at risk. The good citizens who paid out their own money in order to save energy (and reduce the nation's need for more nuclear power stations and the associated ra-diation risks) were, it seemed, suddenly more at risk of dying of another sort of radiation induced illness.

The British Government admitted that the cost of all the work it was recommending was likely to be so great that 100,000 householders might need to hire architects.

But the truth is that the British Government's national ra-don scare seemed to be based on guesswork. Because miners exposed to high radon levels had been found to run an increased risk of lung cancer it was 'assumed' that radon in the home also presented a risk.' Some independent experts disagreed with the Government, claiming that a review of the scientific evidence had revealed 'no direct evidence to incriminate ra-don' and that 'the indirect evidence linking low levels of radon exposure to lung cancer' was 'insufficient to warrant the re-medial action proposed'.

An important American study found no cases of lung can-cer in over 500 miners who had been exposed to vast amounts of radon. In China a study of over 300 cases of lung cancer found no association between lung cancer and radon levels.

In my view the risk posed by radon in the home is probably quite small compared to the dietary risks I have outlined in this book.

APPENDIX ONE

The top ten known causes of cancer

1.	Foods	50%
2.	Tobacco	30%
3.	Alcohol	3%
4.	Radiation (inc X rays)	3%
5.	Sunshine	2%
6	Occupation	2%
7.	Medications	2%
8.	Pollution (air/water)	2%
9.	Passive Smoking	1%
10.	Industrial/household products	1%

These figures are 'estimates' but are based on the available research. I have not included genetic factors or viruses which are known to cause cancer on this table - that is why the total doesn't add up to 100 per cent. The National Academy of Sciences, which concluded that 'cancers of most major sites are influenced by dietary factors' reported that in 1979 researchers using international and intranational comparisons of cancer incidence, the differences between U.S. mortality rates and the lowest reported worldwide mortality rates for each potential cancer site, and results of specific case control studies, had concluded that 'a little more than 40 per cent of cancers in men and almost 60 per cent of cancers in women in the United States could be attributed to dietary factors'. In 1981 it was estimated that dietary modifications might result in a one third reduction in the number of deaths from cancer in the United States - with a 90 per cent reduction in deaths from cancer of the stomach and large bowel; a 50 per cent reduction in deaths from cancers of the endometrium, gallbladder, pancreas and breast; a 20 per cent reduction in deaths from cancers of the lung, larynx, bladder, cervix, mouth, pharynx and oesophagus and a 10 per cent reduction in deaths from other sites.

Many people who are aware that cancer is caused by environmental factors seem to believe that the causes are outside their control - regarding the pollution of air, water and food with chemicals as being the major risk factors. This table clearly shows that food and tobacco are by far the two most important causes of cancer and that, therefore, most people have far more control over their own risk of developing cancer than they realise. It is widely agreed that 80 per cent of all cancers are preventable - using knowledge which we have available at the moment. In other words ignorance (sustained through political and industrial expediency) is responsible for 80 per cent of the millions of deaths caused by cancer each year.

APPENDIX TWO

The early warning signs of cancer

Many cancers are curable - especially if caught early. Here are some of the cancer signs you should watch out for:
● *Cancer of the large bowel:*
change in bowel habits (diarrhoea or constipation), unexplained weight loss, pain, passing blood
● *Cancer of the cervix:*
unexplained bleeding or discharge, pain or bleeding after sex, weight loss
● *Cancer of the breast:*
swelling or lump in breast, bloody discharge from nipple, enlarged glands in armpit, dimpling of the skin of the breast
● *Cancer of the lung:*
persistent bad cough; blood in sputum, chest pain, wheezing, weight loss
● *Cancer of the stomach:*
weight loss, persistent indigestion, vomiting blood, lump in abdomen, feeling full after very small meals
● *Cancer of the liver:*
pain in abdomen, loss of appetite, weight loss, yellow eyes and skin, abdomen swollen
● *Cancer of the ovary:*
irregular periods, hard lump in abdomen, pain during sex, bowel problems, excessive hair growth, voice gets deeper
● *Cancer of the brain:*
headaches, vomiting, visual disturbances, weakness or paralysis, dizziness, fits, memory loss, personality changes
● *Cancer of the skin:*
skin lesion that doesn't heal, bleeds, gets larger, changes shape, size or colour
● *Cancer of the prostate:*
pain, urine retention, difficulty in passing urine
● *Cancer of the testicle:*
swelling in testicle

● *Cancer of the blood (leukaemia):*
tiredness, paleness, bruising, bleeding easily, lots of infections
● *Cancer of the womb*
bleeding after sex, lump felt in abdomen
● *Cancer of the throat:*
hoarseness, lump in throat, difficulty in swallowing, swollen glands in neck

Remember:
A patient with cancer may suffer from one, all or none of these symptoms. These symptom lists are not comprehensive. Patients may suffer from one or more of these symptoms without suffering from cancer. If you are at all worried see your doctor as soon as possible for advice.

APPENDIX THREE

Fighting cancer

Cancer affects every family at some time or other. One in three of us will get it and most people who hear that they have cancer assume the worst.

The commonest and most destructive myth is that cancer always kills. It doesn't. Between a third and half of the people who get cancer recover - usually living long, perfectly healthy, perfectly normal lives. Beating cancer is no longer a miracle. Every year around the world millions of people do it.

The second major myth is that cancer is one disease. It isn't. Cancer is a disease created by deformed or damaged cells. There are scores of different types of cell in your body - bone cells, skin cells, muscle cells and so on and inevitably, therefore, there are scores of different types of cancer. Over 200 in fact.

With so many different types of cancer there are, of course, many different types of treatment. Some cancers can be helped by surgery. Others are best attacked with drugs or radiotherapy.

But there are some things that all cancer patients can do to help themselves:

✓ Make up your mind that you are going to fight.

A study of women with breast cancer showed conclusively that women with a fierce will to live were twice as likely to survive as those who were pessimistic or prepared to abandon themselves to fate.

✓ Spend as much time as you can with people you like and people who make you laugh. There is no doubt now that by watching funny films or reading books that make you chuckle you can help defeat all serious disorders - including cancer.

✓ Assert yourself.If you're in hospital and the doctors and nurses won't tell you things that you want to know make a fuss and make a nuisance of yourself until they answer your questions.People who stand up for themselves stand a much better chance of surviving.

✓ Build up your self confidence. Learn to respect and value yourself. Think of your good qualities and strengths. People who develop and die of cancer often have an unreasonably low opinion of themselves.

✓ Don't be afraid to show your emotions. If you feel angry let your anger out. If you want to cry then cry. Share your emotions with other people. The more you store up your emotions the more damage you'll do to yourself.

✓ Learn to relax yourself. Go off into peaceful, relaxing daydreams whenever stress is building up.

✓ Eat a good, healthy diet containing as much natural food as possible. Fresh fruit and vegetable are much better for you than pre-packed foods.

✓ Join up with other people suffering from the same condition. Your doctors should be able to put your in touch with other local patients who've faced the problem you're facing.

✓ Use the power of your mind to combat your cancer. Think of your cancer cells as bad guys and your body's defence cells as good guys. Imagine your body's defences fighting and destroying frightened cancer cells. This sort of imagery really does work! (For more information see my book 'Mindpower' - which is also published by the European Medical Journal).

✓ Finally, learn as much as you can about your disease. Ignorance breeds fear and anxiety.

APPENDIX FOUR

Breast cancer

The main symptom of breast cancer is usually a lump - most commonly in the upper, outer quarter of the breast. The lump, usually painless, is invariably easier to feel than to see. Other symptoms include changes in the nipple.

● Breast cancer tends to run in families
● Women who have never had children are most at risk of developing breast cancer
● A high protein, high fat diet increases the risk of breast cancer.
● Women who are overweight are more at risk
● A high fibre diet reduces the risk of breast cancer

A few years the standard treatment for breast cancer was complete removal of the breast. Today, however, most surgeons believe that removing just the tumour - rather than the whole breast - produces just as good a survival rate. If a breast cancer is confined to just one lump that has not yet spread then the chances are high that breast removal will not be needed. The patient may also be given drugs and/or radiotherapy.

Many doctors believe that although sophisticated screening systems are now available for testing women's breasts the best way a woman can protect herself is to feel her own breasts regularly - preferably once a week or once a month. Indeed, figures show that despite huge expenditure on screening equipment 90 per cent of breast cancer is discovered by women themselves.

Women are now being officially advised to:

● Check the shape and outline of their breasts for any obvious lumps
● Observe their nipples - looking for changes, bleeding, discharge or inversion
● Physically examine themselves

I suggest that women should examine themselves once a month - preferably just after a menstrual period when their breasts are usually at their softest. Ideally every woman should ask her own family doctor to show her how to examine her breasts.

However, women for whom this is impossible can follow this set plan to reduce the risk of missing any area:

1. Undress to your waist and sit or stand in front of a mirror. Let your hands hang loosely by your sides. Look for any changes in the size or appearance of your breasts or nipples. Look for any puckering or dimpling of the skin and check your nipples for any bleeding or discharge.

2. Lie down. Remember that both breasts will have a soft, general lumpiness because of fat and milk producing glands. Both breasts should feel much the same.

3. Put your left hand under your head. Examine your left breast with your right hand. Use the flat of your fingers not the tips. Begin by examining the inner half of your breast and gradually working your way towards the nipple.

4. Bring your left arm down to your side and examine the other, outer half of your breast in the same way. Feel in your armpit too, looking for any lumps there.

5. Examine your right breast in exactly the same way - but using your left hand.

6. If you find anything unusual or worrying make a mental note of where the lump or change is and make an appointment to see your doctor as soon as possible. In the meantime, try not to keep feeling the lump - it's best to leave it alone.

Finally, remember that few breast lumps are cancerous and that those which are can be treated much more effectively if found early.

How to Conquer Pain

If you suffer from recurrent or persistent pain then you could benefit from reading this invaluable book. It's packed with practical information designed to help you control or banish pain for good. Most exciting of all, it gives details of the many techniques you can use at home to help control and conquer your pain. It describes a small, effective and economical device you can buy which has been shown to relieve pain for 95% of arthritis sufferers. (It can also deal with many other different types of pain too.) There's a very good chance that you've got an excellent source of pain relief in your house, perhaps in your kitchen or in a cupboard somewhere. The book will tell you exactly how to use it against your pain.

"...a brilliant guide, well laid out to explain pain in general, different treatment approaches
and an excellent personal pain management plan"
(The Good Book Guide)

"A clear and helpful handbook for pain sufferers. Perhaps most important of all is the way in which it brings pain down to a manageable level and gives self-help ideas for sufferers"
(The Guardian)

Price £9.95

Published by EMJ Books
Order from Publishing House, Trinity Place, Barnstaple,
Devon EX32 9HJ, England

Also available by Vernon Coleman

Betrayal of Trust

Vernon Coleman catalogues the incompetence and dishonesty of the medical profession and the pharmaceutical industry and explains the historical background to the problems which exist today in the world of healthcare. He shows how drugs are put onto the market without being properly tested, and provides hard evidence for his astonishing assertion that doctors do more harm than good.

"I found (it) so brilliant I could not stop reading it"
(A.P., Luton)

"This blast against the medical establishment certainly makes for a rattling good read"
(The Good Book Guide)

"I urge anyone interested in medicine and the safety of drugs to read Betrayal of Trust"
(Leicester Mercury)

"I feel you should be congratulated for producing something that should be required reading for both consumers and producers of the health
service"
(R.P., Senior Lecturer in Psychology)

Price £9.95

Published by EMJ Books
Order from Publishing House, Trinity Place, Barnstaple,
Devon EX32 9HJ, England

Why Animal Experiments Must Stop

Dr Coleman analyses the pro-vivisection arguments one by one - and destroys them. The moral, ethical, medical and scientific arguments are dealt with and Dr Coleman explains how animal experiments can produce dangerous and misleading information.

Dr Coleman explains that animal experiments are useless today and have always been useless. He goes on to discuss alternatives to animal experiments and offers readers a 10 point action plan with the aim of stopping vivisection for good, so ending one of the world's most barbaric practices.

"A damning indictment of vivisection"
(Animals Today)

"...wonderfully clear and full of good examples"
(M.M., Glasgow)

"... an important book"
(The Vegetarian)

Price £9.95

Published by EMJ Books
Order from Publishing House, Trinity Place, Barnstaple,
Devon EX32 9HJ, England

Bodypower
The secret of self-healing

A new edition of the sensational book which hit the Sunday Times bestseller list and the Bookseller Top Ten Chart.

This international bestseller shows you how you can harness your body's amazing powers to help you cure 9 out of 10 illnesses without seeing a doctor!

The book also covers:

- How your personality affects your health
- How to stay slim for life
- How to improve your eyesight
- How to break bad habits
- How to relax your body and mind
- How to improve your figure
- And much much more!

"Don't miss it. Dr Coleman's theories could change your life"
(Sunday Mirror)

"A marvellously succinct and simple account of how the body can heal itself without resort to drugs"
(The Spectator)

"Could make stress a thing of the past"
(Woman's World)

Price £9.95

Published by EMJ Books
Order from Publishing House, Trinity Place, Barnstaple, Devon EX32 9HJ, England

Also available by Vernon Coleman

People Watching

This fascinating book examines the science and art of people watching. By reading the book and following its advice you will be able to:

- Understand gestures and body language
- Look like a winner
- Negotiate successfully
- Make people like you
- Avoid being manipulated
- Look sexy
- Survive on the street

"The ubiquitous media-doc has done it yet again, this time turning his talents for producing gems of information in rapid-fire sequence to the field of body language and private habits.Once you start to browse you would have to be a hermit not to find it utterly "unputdownable".'
(The Good Book Guide)

"People Watching by Vernon Coleman explains everything you need to know about body language and also how to read individuals by their style of clothes and the colours they wear. There are tips on how to make people like you and how to be a successful interviewee. If you want to look sexy for that special someone or you just want to impress the boss you'll be a winner with this book"
(Evening Telegraph)

Price £9.95

Published by Blue Books
Order from Publishing House, Trinity Place, Barnstaple, Devon EX32 9HJ, England

Toxic Stress
and the Twentieth Century Blues

*'Never have I read a book that is so startlingly true. I was
dumbfounded by your wisdom. You will go down in history as one
of the truly great health reformers of our time'*
(Extracted from a letter to the author)

If you are frustrated, bored, lonely, angry, sad, tired, listless,
frightened, unhappy or tearful then it is possible that you are
suffering from Toxic Stress.

After two decades of research Dr Coleman has come up
with his own antidote to Toxic Stress which he shares with you
in this inspirational book. In order to feel well and happy again
you need to take a close look at your life and put things back in
the right order. Dr Coleman shows you how to value the worthwhile things in life and give less time to things which matter
very little at all. The book contains hundreds of practical tips
on how to cope with the stresses and strains of daily life.

Price £10.95 (hardback)

Published by Chilton Designs Publishers
Order from Publishing House, Trinity Place, Barnstaple,
Devon EX32 9HJ, England

Other books by Vernon Coleman

Food For Thought

Between a third and a half of all cancers may be caused by eating the wrong foods. In this bestselling book Dr Coleman explains which foods to avoid and which to eat to reduce your risk of developing cancer. He also lists foods known to be associated with a wide range of other diseases including Asthma, Gall Bladder Disease, Headaches , Heart Trouble, High Blood Pressure, Indigestion and many more.

Years of research have gone into the writing of this book which explains the facts about mad cow disease, vegetarian eating, microwaves, drinking water, food poisoning, food irradiation and additives. It contains all the information you need about vitamins, carbohydrates, fats and proteins plus a list of 20 superfoods which Dr Coleman believes can improve your health and protect you from a wide range of health problems. The book also includes a "slim-for-life" programme with 48 quick slimming tips to help you lose weight safely and permanently.

" ... a guide to healthy eating which reads like a thriller"
(The Good Book Guide)

"Dr Vernon Coleman is one of our most enlightened, trenchant and sensible dispensers of medical advice"
(The Observer)

Price £9.95
Published by EMJ Books
Order from Publishing House, Trinity Place, Barnstaple, Devon EX32 9HJ, England

Other books by Vernon Coleman

Mindpower

Nothing has the potential to influence your health quite as much as your mind. We've all heard the phrase "you'll worry yourself to death" and scientists have now proved that it is indeed possible for your mind to at least make you ill if not actually kill you. Most doctors around the world now agree that at least 75% of all illnesses can be caused or made worse by stress and/or anxiety. But although your mind can make you ill it can also make you better and has an enormous capacity to heal and cure if only your know how to harness its extraordinary powers and make them work for you - instead of against you!

You can use Mindpower to help you deal with a range of problems including: Anxiety, Depression, Arthritis, Cancer, Asthma, Diabetes,Eczema,Headaches, Heart Disease, High Blood Pressure, Indigestion, Women's Problems, Migraine, Pain,Sleeplessness.

"Dr Coleman's Mindpower is based on an inspiring
message of hope."
(Western Morning News)

"… offers an insight into the most powerful healing agent
in the world - the power of the mind."
(Birmingham Post)

Price £9.95

Published by EMJ Books
Order from Publishing House, Trinity Place, Barnstaple,
Devon EX32 9HJ, England

The Traditional Home Doctor

Vernon Coleman has been writing about health matters for over 25 years and readers have sent him countless thousands of tips and helpful hints. These tips and hints are the sort of information that isn't going to go out of date; they are good, old-fashioned, tried-and-tested methods that have worked for people over the years.

You will find this book a great help the next time you are faced with a family health problem.

The book contains hundreds of easy-to-follow tips on:

- Allergies
- Babies
- Burns
- Colds
- Constipation
- Hay Fever
- Headaches
- Stress
- Sleeplessness
- Tiredness
- Anorexia
- Backache
- Catarrh
- Flu
- Cystitis
- High Blood Pressure
- Indigestion
- Prostate Problems
- Women's Problems
- and much more

Each topic includes lots of tips and hints for solving the problem or reducing troublesome symptoms.

Price £9.95

Published by EMJ Books
Order from Publishing House, Trinity Place, Barnstaple, Devon EX32 9HJ, England

Also available by Vernon Coleman

Alice's Diary

Well over 10,000 delighted readers from around the world have bought this wonderful book which tells of a year in the life of a mixed tabby cat called Alice.

Alice records the year's events and disasters with great humour and insight and at long last gives us a glimpse of what it is really like to be a cat! Delightfully illustrated throughout, this book is an absolute must for animal and cat lovers everywhere.

Price £9.95 (hardback)

Published by Chilton Designs Publishers
Order from Publishing House, Trinity Place, Barnstaple,
Devon EX32 9HJ, England

The Man Who Inherited a Golf Course

The title says it all! Trevor Dukinfield, the hero of the story, wakes up one morning to discover that he is the owner of his very own golf club - fairways, bunkers, clubhouse and all. It has been left to him in his uncle's will, but there are some very strange conditions attached to his inheritance. To keep the club he must win an important match. The only snag is that he has never played a round of golf in his life.

Price £12.95 (hardback)

Published by Chilton Designs Publishers
Order from Publishing House, Trinity Place, Barnstaple,
Devon EX32 9HJ, England

Also available by Vernon Coleman

The Bilbury Chronicles

A young doctor arrives to begin work in the small village of Bilbury. This picturesque hamlet is home to some memorable characters who have many a tale to tell, and Vernon Coleman weaves together a superb story full of humour and anecdotes. The Bilbury books will transport you back to the days of old-fashioned, traditional village life where you never needed to lock your door, and when a helping hand was only ever a moment away. The first novel in the series.

"I am just putting pen to paper to say how very much I enjoyed The Bilbury Chronicles. I just can't wait to read the others."
(Mrs K., Cambs)

"...a real delight from cover to cover. As the first in a series it holds out the promise of entertaining things to come"
(Daily Examiner)

"The Bilbury novels are just what I've been looking for. They are a pleasure to read over and over again"
(Mrs C., Lancs)

Price £12.95 (hardback)

Published by Chilton Designs Publishers
Order from Publishing House, Trinity Place, Barnstaple, Devon EX32 9HJ, England

Also available by Vernon Coleman

Bilbury Grange

The second novel in the Bilbury series sees the now married doctor moving into his new home - a vast and rambling country house in desperate need of renovation. With repair bills soaring and money scarce, the doctor and his new wife look for additional ways to make ends meet. Another super novel in this series - perfect for hours of escapism!

"I have just finished reading Bilbury Grange. I found the book to be brilliant. I felt as though I was part of the community. Please keep me informed of any more in this excellent series."
(Mr C, Cleethorpes)

"A wonderful book for relaxing and unwinding. Makes you want to up roots and move to the rural heartland."
(Lincolnshire Echo)

"For sheer relaxing pleasure here's another witty tale from the doctor whose prolific writings are so well known."
(Bookshelf)

Price £12.95 (hardback)

Published by Chilton Designs Publishers
Order from Publishing House, Trinity Place, Barnstaple, Devon EX32 9HJ, England

The Bilbury Revels

Disaster strikes in this the third Bilbury novel when a vicious storm descends on the village. The ensuing snow storm cuts off the village and blankets the whole area in a deep carpet of snow. Much damage is done to the village as a result of the storm and the locals band together to undertake the repair work. Money, as ever, is tight and fund-raising is of prime importance. Money-spinning suggestions are sought and so the idea of the Revels is born - a week of fun and festivities to raise the money needed to repair the local schoolteacher's cottage.

Price £12.95 (hardback)

Published by Chilton Designs Publishers
Order from Publishing House, Trinity Place, Barnstaple,
Devon EX32 9HJ, England

Bilbury Pie

A delightful collection of short stories based in and around this fictional Devon village.

Every community has its characters and Bilbury is no exception! Thumper Robinson is the local "jack the lad" and Pete is the taxi driver, shop owner, funeral director and postman all rolled into one. Patchy Fogg dispenses advice on antiques to anyone who will listen and Dr Brownlow is the eccentric and rather elderly, retired local doctor

Price £9.95(hardback)

Published by Chilton Designs Publishers
Order from Publishing House, Trinity Place, Barnstaple,
Devon EX32 9HJ, England